From Couch Potato to Weekend Athlete

By Brian Borgford

For Tony and Cam
Who inspired my journey and still do.

My Journey

If you've ever had a fleeting desire to learn how to run, this book is for you. If you've ever contemplated running in a ten-kilometre race but opted out because it seemed too daunting, this book is for you. If running a marathon or doing a triathlon ever crossed your mind but you shoved it out, thinking, "No, not me," then this book is for you. Or if you just want to lose weight and get healthy, there is motivation for you in these pages.

Follow my inspirational journey from being a fat, middle-aged suburbanite to running races and competing in triathlons. If I can do it, you can do it.

This book is not meant to tell you what to do, but rather show how one man faced the improbable and turned it into reality. Read about my metamorphosis and personal experiences in accomplishing what I never thought was possible. Learning about my journey may help you map your own voyage to be the person you never thought you could be. Physical health and fitness are the visible benefits, but the effect on the psyche and personal confidence supersedes all other benefits. It's all there for the taking, by anyone. As Nike says, "Just do it."

The book includes plans for how you too can become athletic, healthy, and fit, and perhaps even participate in those weekend events you see around your community or beyond. You can find many how-to books on various activities, but this is one of the few stories that details "how I did it," complete with specific experiences and actual, rather than proposed, training plans.

You don't need to follow my exact path; you can reach your peak or pinnacle at any place along your own path. The important thing is to choose to start. After that you have a wealth of positive choices.

Give it a tri (try?). What have you got to lose? You may even gain a new perspective on life, as did I.

In The Beginning

If something is worth doing, it is worth doing to excess. It took me a long time to realize that I live by this unspoken motto.

I was a latecomer to drinking and smoking, not really getting started until my late teens while attending university, but I managed to make up for lost time, ensuring that no one could consume more alcohol or smoke more cigarettes than I could.

By my mid-twenties, I was married with two sons. I could sit down on a Friday evening with the colour TV showing one football game, a little black-and-white TV at my side showing a hockey game, and the Saskatchewan Roughriders football game blaring in my earphones from my transistor radio. At my side was a twelve-pack of beer that would hopefully last me through the sporting events and an ashtray big enough to hold the butts from at least one pack of cigarettes.

Life was good. I worked hard, I played hard, and I even had time for my young boys, who were now getting active with school and sports.

I began to realize that my lifestyle was on full display for my sons, and that I had come to this lifestyle by modelling my behaviours after that of my family: my father, mother, and, even more so, my much older brothers.

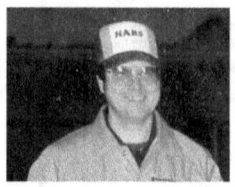

Me before I started my journey

As much as I was enjoying my life, I knew it wasn't what I wished for my sons to emulate.

In late 1982, I made the rash decision to give up smoking. Having done so a couple of times in the past, once even for two years, I didn't announce this decision to anyone for fear that I might fail again. I didn't pick some magic date, like my thirtieth birthday or New Year. I just did it one day. I got up and said to myself, "I'll try one day without a smoke." And then I tried another and another. This attempt at quitting was much tougher than my previous endeavours, and I had to work at it to keep from falling back into the habit. I needed a substitute for cigarettes, so I picked barbequed peanuts as my crutch. And I hadn't given up drinking yet.

The results: I gave up smoking for good. However, with the extra snacks and extra alcohol that came from not having to alternate between puffs and gulps, I ballooned to over two hundred pounds, when my frame suggests an upper limit of one hundred seventy-five pounds.

I was no longer modelling the disgusting behaviour of smoking, but my drinking had increased to the point where I wondered if I was becoming addicted. I didn't think so, but it nagged at me. I occasionally would cut back to a social level of drinking, but my unspoken motto always got the better of me—do it to excess. Why have two beers when you can have six or eight?

Other contributing factors to my drinking were my work and travel. I spent much of my time on airplanes, where alcohol was served free and freely. My workmates who travelled with me all drank, and although smoking was on the decline among the business travellers, drinking was still at its peak. This was the era of the two-martini lunch and after-work drinking binges, especially when travelling to another city and living the hotel life.

Early in 1985 I decided to do something about my drinking. I was determined to become a social drinker and deal with my weight problem, which caused me to look like some freak I couldn't recognize. I also needed to know if I had a dependency on alcohol.

I began swimming at lunchtime. I worked my way up to the point where I could swim non-stop for one thousand to fifteen hundred metres. At the same time, I forced myself to keep my drinking to a one- or two-beer maximum at any function, proving to myself that I was not an alcoholic.

I even started to play racquetball with some workmates to supplement my swimming. I did very little to change my eating habits, but the altered lifestyle seemed to have an unplanned effect on my meal patterns. I began to lose weight—only a little at first, but it was noticeable.

I used swimming as my main form of exercise, not wanting to embrace other forms of weight control, such as running, that so many people were taking up during the mid-eighties fitness craze. I could usually find a swimming pool, even during my business travel, as the hotels had pools I could use.

During this time, I put forth a proposal to my employer to take a two-year leave of absence to obtain my master of business administration (MBA). With this request finally approved, my job as controller for the company was posted, leading many to speculate that my overwhelming weight loss was due to illness and that I was dying.

Attending a family wedding in Minneapolis, I stayed at a hotel that didn't have a swimming pool. I was petrified. I had become addicted to my swimming and was getting used to being able to see my feet again without my belly blocking the view. Flipping through the hotel literature for directions to the nearest pool, I saw some information on running. The brochure had a couple of premarked running routes, one of which was a mile long.

I donned my court shoes I had brought along just in case I got a chance to play some racquetball, and I did a one-mile run/walk. At the end of this twenty-minute outing, I felt a twinge of pride at having actually run much of the distance. As a youth in high school, I was relegated to the "also-ran" group due to my limited athletic ability, so I had always avoided running as a form of exercise. I recalled an instance only a few years earlier of gasping for air as I tried to catch an escaping bus, forcing me to wait another half hour for the next one.

The following day I did it again, running farther and walking less. After the wedding events—where I decided to not even be a social drinker and opted instead for a night of sipping water—I moved to my brother's house for the remainder of my stay in Minneapolis. His home was in the middle of a local running route, which included a hill leading up to the house. I gave it a try and ran the whole way—almost three kilometres. I was now a runner, and my motto would be applied to a new excessive habit.

Returning home after the wedding festivities, I began a daily running regime while still hanging on to my daily swims. I arose each morning before 5:00 a.m. to run unseen through our neighbourhood and also made my noon jaunts over to the Lawson Aquatic Centre for my fifteen-hundred-metre swims.

I was now a mere shadow of my former self, having dropped forty pounds in less than three months. Smoking had ceased three years earlier, and I was now a social drinker, confirming my status of "not an alcoholic."

As my departure for my MBA was imminent, rumours of my health ran rampant at the office.

Business Travel

On one business trip, Ken, a co-worker, and I were going to a training session in Montreal and stopped for a couple days in Mississauga for some business. We had been drinking buddies on many previous business trips, but I told him this time we would be saints and not drink and exercise daily instead. Ken resented my altered behaviours but participated anyway. I got him up grumbling for early morning runs, and we went to the gym, not the bar, after work. But in Montreal we had a major slip-up. I planned on running in the mornings and going to the gym after the training session, but somehow we ended up taking advantage of the Montreal nightlife. For the first time in ages, I went well beyond my social drinking limit and we got plastered, not realizing that the bars in Montreal don't close—not at any sane hour anyway. In spite of being still inebriated, I got up at five in the morning for a run before our training started. I donned my shorts and running shoes and sat on the edge of the bed. Next thing I knew, I woke up and was half an hour late for my seminar. I rushed to get ready and joined the group, albeit late, but I still beat Ken by half an hour. I vowed never to repeat this lifestyle infraction.

Setback

A major event changed my daily pattern. The Lawson Aquatic Centre was closing for a month for renovations and I would lose my noon swim time. But not to worry, I could run in the morning and then join the noon running crowd, now that I was a real runner rather than a fat, middle-aged suburbanite. I was running fifty to eighty kilometres each week. That is excessive, even for an experienced marathoner.

On a noon run with Terry, one of my workmates, I felt a strange sensation in my left knee. I kept running, but by half-way I could barely move my leg and told Terry I would meet him back at the office. I hobbled for a while, getting angry at my bad fortune. I forced a run for about five hundred metres before realizing I couldn't do it and hobbled the rest of the way back to our office building. After limping through the shower and struggling back to my office, I had to call Marlene, my wife, to come and take me to the doctor. "Oh, and by the way," I told her, "bring mom's old cane along."

She met me at my office, and I had to use the cane to make my way to the car. We went to Dr. Thakrar, who prescribed some oral anti-inflammatory and no running. I could only hobble with the cane, so running wasn't in my current vocabulary, but I had become so addicted to running that I was anxious to get this problem behind me. Dr. Thakrar had first diagnosed chondromalacia (a snapping of a tendon against the back of the knee cap), and then settled on a form of bursitis (like tennis elbow, only on the knee). The problem was that the connective tissue between the tendon and the bone was damaged and had become inflamed.

Days turned into a week, and then two weeks, and into a third week. My hobbling had progressed to a shuffle, but there was still little improvement in my condition. Dr. Thakrar gave me even stronger anti-inflammatory drugs, but there was still no real improvement. With almost three weeks of no running, I was getting concerned that I might not be able to call myself a runner. After pleading with Dr. Thakrar to do something, he referred me to a specialist, a young, cocksure, arrogant runt of a doctor who seemed to specialize in my type of ailment. He asked me a few questions, but very few. The question I recall best was when he asked how many miles I ran each week. I replied, "Fifty miles per week," which is what I had been doing with my twice-daily runs, a training regime that any athlete would tell you is stupid, especially for a rookie runner. The brash doctor exclaimed, "What? Are you a government worker?"

With a brief visual examination and the answers to his few questions, he made his diagnosis and was ready to move to the cure. He pulled out a needle bigger than any I had seen since I'd gotten penicillin shots in the butt as a child with rheumatic fever. He filled the vial attached to the needle with some kind of fluid. Although I was shocked by what was transpiring so quickly, I put my trust in this little fellow to cure me. He pushed the huge needle into the knee, right at the center of the pain and discomfort. I thought I would leap out the window; the flow of the liquid into my knee caused a sensation bordering between excruciating pain and death. The three seconds that it took to expel the liquid into my knee felt like hours.

"OK, done. Now no running for at least a couple days," the doctor told me. I was sure I would never walk again, let alone run, so this instruction seemed redundant. I stood up to see if I could put any pressure on my leg after the knee being filled with what turned out to be cortisone and found I could stand with minimal discomfort. I was able to walk out of the clinic using the stairs as opposed to shuffling into the elevator as I had when I entered. By the time I reached the car I felt like I could actually run. In a flash I realized why so many athletes used cortisone as a miracle cure to keep their careers going. The doctor had warned me on my way out to never have another cortisone treatment in that area for the rest of my life. It provided a quick cure, but overuse would eat away at every piece of tissue around the joint and render it useless. I was ecstatic to be cured.

I followed the doctor's instructions by waiting a few days before starting a slow running regime. Then I gradually picked up the pace and distance at a rate recommended in the many editions of *Runner's World* magazine I had taken to reading. I vowed to never let my excesses put me out of commission again. I was more addicted to running than I ever was to alcohol.

Hockey

The previous winter, when I was still overweight and a heavy drinker, had been my third season with an over-thirty hockey team. I wasn't much of a hockey player, but my social habits made me a perfect fit for all other team activities, especially the postgame drinking binge in the dressing room at midnight. My teammates, all of them heavy drinkers and most of them smokers, had tolerated my dropping of the smoking habit. It had actually made me a better player on the ice, but that didn't take much. I could still out-drink most of them in the postgame activities. Entering this new season, I was now almost a non-drinker, relegating myself to only one or two beers when drinking. After the games, I mostly just drank water.

The only time I revisited my old habits was after one rare Saturday afternoon game. Because the dressing room was needed after our match, we retired to the Hot Spot restaurant, one of our regular haunts for pizza and beer. I had more than my now usual one or two beers; it was actually closer to six glasses of draught beer. When I came home, my sons commented on my strange behaviour and said that I was acting silly. They had become used to seeing me without the effects of alcohol. That was the last drop of alcohol I ever drank. I had proved I didn't need it and didn't enjoy small quantities, so I quit forever. My brother Alvin would say, "This is my brother Brian. He doesn't drink. He quit and didn't even need to go to meetings."

Moving to London

I continued my recreational running, trying to avoid any excesses that might result in injury, got back into my swimming when the Lawson reopened, and started thinking about supplementing it all with some cycling. I fixed up an old ten-speed I had purchased at a garage sale and went on a few bike rides. In the back of my mind I started thinking, "Swim, bike, run—triathlon? Maybe. Not bloody likely, but who knows?"

When I moved my family to London, Ontario, to pursue my MBA while on a two-year paid leave of absence, I vowed to keep up my exercise. I had worked hard to shed my former couch-potato existence, and I never wanted to go back. The university was about eight to ten kilometres from our home by road, but using some shortcuts while running or biking, I found a five-kilometre route. I used a mix of biking and running as my form of transportation to and from the university, leaving our only car available for Marlene. The university had a great fitness facility with a large pool, and I was able to keep up an almost daily swimming routine to supplement my running and biking. I stayed fit during my entire MBA program, and that likely helped me maintain my sanity with the torturous coursework. I found I carried much less stress than my classmates, and I attributed much of that to my healthy lifestyle. I even made the dean's honour list.

I kept formulating goals in my mind and mentally committed to three activities sometime in the next few years. I wanted to run a ten-kilometre race, do a marathon, and compete in an Olympic distance triathlon.

An opportunity to knock one of those off my list presented itself while I was still in London, during the break between my first and second years of the MBA program. I wrote about this experience, my first ten-kilometre race, many years later, after I took up the hobby of writing. Here is that story, which was entered (unsuccessfully) in a writing contest to produce a story without using *the* anywhere in the narrative.

My First Ten-Kilometre Race

A sign hit me as I left, after my workout. I didn't normally look at bulletin boards, but a bright blue sign jumped out at me.

10 kilometre race
Strathroy Road Runners Club
Saturday, June 10
Contact...

Ever since I'd started running two years earlier, I had set three goals for myself. Run a 10K race, run a marathon, and compete in a triathlon.

Was it now time to start on my list? I was sure I could run ten kilometres. I normally ran five to eight kilometres every day, but I had never actually done an entire 10K distance. But in Strathroy, who would even know me? It was perfect. If I did it, I could brag about it. If I couldn't complete it or if I performed poorly, who would know?

I didn't tell Marlene or my boys. I got up early Saturday morning before anyone was out of bed. A 7:00 a.m. start and an hour's drive. I wanted to be there in lots of time to register, so I left at 5:00 a.m. and was there by 6:00 a.m.

There wasn't much of a line-up when I arrived, but I felt intimidated. I had never been in a race, and all of these fit athletes were comparing times and placements. I didn't even know what a good time would be for a 10K distance. I knew I ran about eight minutes per mile or five minutes per kilometre. I didn't want to be last.

I wore my New Balance 750s, which were a standard runner. Others had some hi-tech lightweight racing flats. But I did notice a few plain runners like mine. By start time there were about two hundred runners gathering around a crowded start line. An organizer shouted over a loudspeaker that racing would start in two minutes. My heart was pounding like I had already run three kilometres. I was scared and all alone. Everyone else seemed to know each other.

"On your mark, get set—" *Boom!* exploded a starter's pistol and runners bolted. I pumped my feet and arms as fast as I could to keep from falling behind before even starting. Leaders were hundreds of metres in front of me, but I was in a crowd keeping pace. I wasn't falling behind. And there were dozens or more behind me.

I pushed my heart rate as high as I could and tried to hold it. At three kilometres I saw a fit young fellow limping, coming toward us. He had come up lame and was pulling out. *That happens? I hope not to me.*

I reached five kilometres, halfway. I was hanging in. I was puffing hard but not fading. And I was still in a pack of other runners.

By eight kilometres some of my pack was falling behind. I was actually beating people. Nine-kilometre mark—only one kilometre to go. I poured it on. My competitive nature started to emerge. I left my pack behind as I picked up my pace for a home-stretch run.

I finished and clicked my Timex running watch. It read 42:55. I didn't know if that was good or bad, but I felt great. My race was over, and I was floating. I was lighter than air. I had done it, and I felt no pain.

I walked and jogged to cool down. It was effort-less. I jogged back. There were still people coming in and lots of people yet to finish. More than fifteen minutes passed before all runners finished. I must have done OK.

Organizers announced that breakfast was being served. I hadn't paid any attention, but my race en-try included a pancake breakfast. So I lined up to eat. I was so excited I wanted to talk to someone about my experience. But I knew no one. I tried to strike up a conversation, but everyone was wrapped up in his or her own stories and friends. I sat at a picnic table with some strangers while I gobbled my pancakes. I got some casual talk from a few, but mostly I sat alone.

Organizers started to hand out awards and draw prizes. I got neither. Then everyone began clamoring around a bulletin board. Results were posted.

I pushed my way in front to get a look. Although I didn't win anything, I saw I finished thirty-second out of over two hundred runners. I was far from last.

I hopped in my car for a sixty-minute drive home. I still felt like I was floating on air. Marlene asked where I had been. She'd woken up and found me and our car gone. She was worried. I couldn't stop talking about my experience. I was still pumped.

By midafternoon I was starting to fade. I lay down for a nap and never woke up until Sunday morning.

I could now strike item one off my list.

The Start of Racing— Season 1

I kept my exercise routine front and centre in my life, much like a religion. Having received my MBA and an award for making the dean's honour list while being a runner, I attributed much of my success at school to the discipline imposed by fitting a solid exercise regime into an already heavy academic schedule. I re-entered the workforce after my degree feeling like I could conquer the world.

I read books and magazines on running and even started to pick up the occasional *Triathlete* magazine. One book on running, a paperback with a green cover, became my bible. I would talk to anyone who would listen and even to those who didn't want to listen. I was always able to locate other runners who would share running stories. I became a regular with the noon running crowd at work, doing the Wascana Lake circuit in Regina.

I had only participated in one race in my life, my ten-kilometre effort in Strathroy, Ontario, but that was about to change. It was the summer of 1990. Our company entered a team in the annual Corporate Challenge, which consisted of a series of silly physical events. However it did have a twenty-kilometre race as part of the activities. Each team was to supply four runners, each of whom would run the five-kilometre loop of Wascana Lake. Being an avid runner, I was approached for the running team and I accepted. I completed the five-kilome-tre loop in just over twenty-one minutes, making me the sec-ond fastest runner on the team, behind only Don, a co-worker and fellow runner, who was just under twenty-one minutes. I was ecstatic, and for the second time in my life experienced the floating sensation known as the runner's high. It's like a drug, and it is addicting. I knew I had to do more.

Some of the noon-hour runners started talking about an upcoming event in Regina, the fifteen-kilometre Buffalothon race. I had only raced as far as ten kilometres and had really not done any running beyond eight to ten kilometres, but I was sure I could do it. And I did. My second race that year saw me finish the fifteen kilometres in sixty-six minutes. Again, I experienced the runner's high and had no fatigue or aches and pains. I needed more.

A few weeks later I went to Saskatoon to participate in a twenty-kilometre race, finishing in less than eighty-eight minutes. The end of the summer of 1990 saw the Brooks Downtown Dash, a ten-kilometre race attended by thousands. I completed this race in about forty-two minutes, faster than my Strathroy time. I had completed four races that summer and could hardly wait for the next season.

Season 2

I continued my running and swimming all winter. I also purchased an inexpensive exercise bike to ride at home, to keep up my cycling during the winter, just in case I got the chance to do a triathlon. Early in 1991 I picked up a racing schedule from one of the sports shops. It had all the dates and times for the Timex Road Race Series in Saskatchewan. I recalled from a few years earlier, when I had just started running, that Norm, an avid runner and one of my staff, had thrown one of these annual schedules on my desk. He'd heard that I had just started running. I'm sure he did this as a smart-ass move, thinking, "Here, fat guy, why don't you try some real running instead of that jogging stuff?" I'd brushed it off then, but now I was ready to look at the schedule seriously.

I mapped out several races that fit around my travel plans and started running some of them. I knew I would never win any races, especially in my competitive under-forty category, but I loved being in the racing environment and feeling the rush when I crossed the finish line.

Having a couple of ten-kilometre races under my belt by June, and getting closer to the forty-one-minute mark, I happened to see a sign for a triathlon posted on the bulletin board of the Lawson Aquatic Centre, where I still swam. I stared at it, but walked away. The next time I went for a swim, I made sure I had a pen and paper and copied down all the particulars, including the name and phone number of the race organizer in Saskatoon, where the race would be held the following Saturday, in early June of 1991.

In the meantime, I had been in constant contact with Hans, a co-worker in our Mississauga office who had been competing in triathlons for years. I wanted to know everything about triathlons and grilled him every time I could. He informed me of a race coming up in Milton, Ontario, which coincided with a business trip I had planned around that time. I told him if he could locate a bike for me to use, I might consider doing that as my first triathlon. Triathletes love to get people hooked on their sport, and he went to work to make sure I did that race, including tracking down an excellent bike for me to use. The distances were a one-kilometre swim, thirty-two-kilometre bike ride, and an eight-kilometre run, not quite Olympic distance but getting close. I couldn't turn him down now, so I told him to sign me up—I was now committed to trying the second item on my list, a triathlon.

Saskatoon Sprint Triathlon

I was scared. Could I do it? Would I panic? What about an open water swim?

When I looked at the particulars of the Saskatoon race, it included an Olympic distance (1.5 km swim, 40 km bike, 10 km run), but it also included a sprint distance consisting of a five-hundred-metre pool swim, twenty-kilometre bike, and a five-kilometre run. This would be a perfect warm-up and confidence builder for my race in Ontario the next month. I phoned Ron, the race organizer, for more information. I actually had all the information I needed; what I was really looking for was some encouragement. My stomach was in knots thinking about doing my first triathlon in less than a week. Ron gave me all the details, which were the same as what was on the poster.

Then I told him this would be my first triathlon and asked if he had any tips. I think this line of questioning caught him off guard, as he seemed to stumble through some generic advice: start slow, don't overdo it, get your bearings on the bike, ease up as you are coming off the bike route, and so on. It wasn't particularly helpful, but, again, I was really looking for encouragement. He said I could register over the phone and pay on race day. So I was in—only a few days until my first triathlon and the second item on my to-do list.

Marlene and I drove up to Saskatoon on Saturday, the day before the Sunday race. I don't think I could have handled arriving on race day just before the race. We drove to the race venue, an indoor fifty-metre pool. I drove the bike route to get an idea where I was going and also scoped out the running route as best as I could.

I arrived early for race registration and to get set up. I had done some research on what it was like to set up and do transitions in a triathlon, but seeing it in real life was intimidating. I set my bike up on one of the bike racks. I had a used bike I had bought while in London, and it still had the rack over the rear wheel where I used to carry my panniers. I started to shiver as I watched other competitors set up their transition areas. The bikes were unlike any I had ever seen. They were sleek and light; most of them had tri-bars (a piece of equipment that clip on your handle bars allowing you to lean your forearms on) for speed. Many had drinking systems that avoided the clumsy use of water bottles. All had cycling shoes and clipless pedals. I had my running shoes that slipped into a metal cage; it was completely obsolete equipment.

The competitors looked like athletes, some with trisuits (a one-piece outfit for swimming, biking and running), all with cycling pants. Many set up buckets and towels near their bikes where they could wash their feet before they donned their cycling shoes. I started to wonder, *What am I doing here? I don't belong.* But I persevered and tried to soak in as much data as I could since in a few weeks I would be doing this again in Milton.

I met up with Denard, the husband of Marlene's cousin. I had known Denard for many years, but had forgotten that he did triathlons. He was competing in the Olympic distance event, so he was busy getting himself ready for the race, but I was able to soak in a few tips from him.

The race organizers called all the competitors together to bark out the final instructions and route directions and any hazards to watch out for. Then we were all sent into the indoor fifty-metre pool to get ready to start the race. I wasn't too worried about a five-hundred-metre swim, as I had been doing almost fifteen hundred every day anyway. But now to do it with other racers felt daunting. We were to start the swim in five-second intervals and were told that passing needed to be done on the return lap, as they had the lanes set up for maximum efficiency and capacity. My heart thumped as I awaited my turn to start the swim, watching others in my lane depart. Then I was sent off.

"Go!" shouted the race marshal for our lane, and I took off at full tilt. Although I had done lots of swimming and at long distances, I had never raced before. I started out with my head in the water and only took a breath after almost ten strokes to maximize my speed. In my normal swimming I took a breath every second or third stroke. What I found out was that you need much more oxygen when you are racing, and holding your breath that long can be fatal in a race. After my second breath, almost twenty strokes, I could hardly breathe and thought I was going to faint. I panicked, wondering if I was going to have to pull out before I even started. Then I slowed my stroke and reverted to my normal breathing pattern and was able to complete the five hundred metres and gratefully exit the water to get ready for my bike ride. I survived the swim ordeal.

My first ever transition wasn't perfect, but it was OK. I only had to put on my runners, a T-shirt, and helmet and I was on my way. The bike ride went smoothly, and I even passed a few people on the route. Finishing comfortably, all I had to do was toss my helmet, park the bike, and start to run. I was in my element with the running, passing many people along the way. I felt the runner's high as I crossed the finish line with lots of extra energy. I knew I could easily handle longer distances.

At the social and awards luncheon after the race I sat with Denard and pulled as much triathlon information from him that I could. I was impressed when he was called up as the second-place finisher of the over-forty masters category of the Olympic distance event; he had just turned forty that year and was one year older than me. Of course, I won nothing in the sprint event and was not expecting to. However I did win a draw prize, my first. It was a pair of clipless pedals, but of a variety that even Denard had never seen. I discovered that many of the better prizes were actually slow-moving or obsolete stock from various sporting goods stores. I later bought a used pair of biking shoes and tried these pedals out for a while, but discarded them once I learned why they were obsolete and a pain to use.

I pored over the results printout distributed to the participants. Denard was only seconds behind the first-place finisher in his category, Murray. The third place was considerably behind the two of them. I placed a respectable fifth place in my category in the sprint event. But some quick math showed me that if I had been competing in the Olympic distance event and could maintain the same pace as I had in the sprint event, I could have been the third-place finisher in the over-forty group—if I were over forty, which I would be next year.

I left the event with a combination of pride and elation for what I had just finished, but also anxiety about doing the Milton event the next month.

I continued doing the local running events and getting marginally faster with each one, but I was stuck at a certain pace, about four and a quarter minutes per kilometre. Don, who had become a regular running buddy of mine, and I seesawed back and forth as to who would beat the other at any given race, but there were only a few seconds difference between us.

Milton Triathlon

Next up was my trip to Ontario and my second triathlon. Hans was a big help in getting me mentally ready and providing me with a borrowed bike. He even went on a training ride with me to let me get a feel for the roads near the race site. The borrowed bike was a Cadillac compared to my too-small Bianchi, and I realized that if I were to keep at this sport, I would need to upgrade.

Hans was not doing the race himself, opting instead to be a race marshal. So he was on hand before the race, which was comforting to me as I was even more intimidated than in my previous race. In Saskatoon there were only about a hundred and fifty competitors between the two events, however the Milton race had several hundred in just one event. The transition zone was filled with even more hi-tech bikes than I saw in the previous race with some shapes that barely resembled a bike. Some of the helmets looked like they came from outer space. My borrowed bike, as good as it was, still paled in comparison to the other gear in the transition zone.

This was to be my first open water swim. We had to walk to one end of a small lake and then swim to the other end where we would exit the water and enter the transition zone. I started to panic about the swim, recalling my last fiasco at the start of the event. I was ready to chicken out when I saw most of the racers donning wetsuits. I only had some cycling shorts, which doubled as swim trunks. Why did you need a wetsuit? Did they know something I didn't?

I sought out Hans to ask him about this turn of events. He said that many triathletes use wetsuits whenever the water temperature allows, but that the water was warm enough to swim without. That calmed me somewhat, but I was still nervous about the swim.

When the horn signaled the start of the swim, everyone rushed down the beach, pushing and shoving their way until they could fall forward in the water and get their arms rotating. I joined the crowd, regretting my placement in the middle where I was jostled, had my goggles kicked off my face, and felt elbows jabbing at me as I tried to gain some motion in the splashing turmoil all around me. I got my goggles positioned back on my face and was able to separate from the main pack of swimmers, probably because I was falling behind. It was the longest twenty-two minutes I could remember. I had expected to be well under twenty minutes based on my pool times, but the crowded open water swim was an experience that required tactics that come with experience, which I didn't have yet.

I was elated to be out of the water and heading for the bike. The bike ride was heaven compared to the swim. I even found myself passing some of the hi-tech bikes with my borrowed bike. But there were people passing me as well. Given that the race started in waves, some of those passing by me or others could have been due to different start times. One humbling experience was watching an older gentleman on a triathlon bike breeze by me like I was standing still. It looked like this fellow was at least twenty, if not twenty-five, years older than me. I actually enjoyed the bike ride more than I ever expected to and had no trouble making the transition to the run, where I felt at home.

The run was an out and back with a long steep climb up a hill where we turned around at the top and returned the same way we came. I relished the climb that allowed me to pass many runners on my way up, and I felt like I was floating for the second half, which was all downhill. I finished the eight kilometres in thirty-four minutes. The runner's high followed me across the finish line.

Hans was not able to stay past the end of the race, which left me with no one I knew to share my exhilarating experience.

I attended the postrace social having little interaction with the other competitors, who all seemed to know one another. I did get to sit beside the older fellow who had passed me on the bike. He was in his mid-sixties and in great shape. We talked for a few minutes when he excused himself. He said that racing made him tired and he needed to close his eyes for a while. He sat with his back propped up against a tree and nodded off.

My second triathlon was in the bag, and I felt great. I wanted more.

Regina Beach Triathlon

Denard had told me about a triathlon coming up in Regina Beach, only about a half hour drive from Regina. It was more or less an Olympic distance race, except the bike was forty-six kilometres in order to take in the Lumsden Hill. Most triathlons alter their courses based on the terrain, water, and roads. I had now done two triathlons, but neither was the Olympic distance, so I felt compelled to do this one to make sure I could stroke *triathlon* off my list.

I still had no wetsuit and most of the racers put one on for the swim. But this time I took note of the many people who did not wear a wetsuit and I felt I should be OK. It was July in Saskatchewan and the water was warm enough.

As I racked my bike and saw all of the better bikes around me, my intimidation factor was now lower. I now felt more embarrassed because of my old blue bike with the red rack still on the back. This was a much smaller and less intimidating crowd than I had faced in Milton, so I was feeling more at ease with the setting. Having two previous events under my belt was a confidence builder.

However, as the race director announced the route, my heart sank. I realized that we had to swim across the lake, not out and back or in a triangle or circle. They were taking us by boat to the far side, and we had to swim back. It was labelled as one and one-half kilometres, but when you see that all in one straight line, it looks like ten miles. Denard was in this race as well, but his nemesis, Murray, was not. So Denard was looking forward to what he called a hollow victory. I also struck up a conversation with another experienced triathlete, Mike, on the boat ride over. This was a much friendlier crowd than I had experienced in the other races. I asked Mike how long he expected to take to cross the lake and he replied about half an hour. I felt better knowing that his expected time was near what I hoped to do for fifteen hundred metres.

I had been overwhelmed enough with the one-kilometre swim in Milton in a small, shallow lake, but this swim, across a much bigger body of water, really scared me. There was little chance of bailing out in midswim, although they did have support boats following the swimmers. Once on the opposite side, I could not see the end of the swim route where we could exit the water. How would I find my way? There were only a few dozen racers, and I was sure I would be separated from most of them by the time we got a couple hundred metres, and I couldn't figure out how to keep my bearings. Mike helped by pointing out a building on the opposite side to use as a landmark, but once we got in the water, I couldn't see anything on the other shore. So I just kept swimming, trying to keep other swimmers in sight, but losing ground, or more accurately, losing water.

I saw a boat on my right side, so I thought I would use one of the support boats as a guide and made sure I swam close to it. It turned out to be a fishing boat, not a support boat, and it kept moving away from me as I approached. I ended up several hundred metres off course. When I finally did exit the water, I had to run a long way to find the transition zone, but I did and got on my bike for the second leg.

The route out of Regina Beach to Highway 11, where the bulk of the bike course took place, included a five-hundred-metre-long hill right out of the water. I had little experience with hill climbing and I was scared I would have to get off and push my bike up and look like a real loser. I stayed on the bike and pumped with all my might and made it to the top. This would be the longest ride I had ever done. I carried two water bottles on my bike for hydration, but I made sure that I took in lots of water before the race. Big mistake. Water in means water out. I wasn't ten kilometres into the ride when I realized I had to pee, and pee badly. I tried to think of something else as I pedaled as hard as I could, but the sensation wouldn't go away. I recalled hearing about the long-distance randonneur cyclists who urinated while on long rides. I realized that there was no one near me on the bike, so I thought I would give it a try. No luck. There was no way my body was going to let me pee while riding, so I just held on, thinking I might have to take a longer transition to relieve myself.

Although the first half of the bike was a breeze, the cycling ordeal lasted even longer than I expected. At the turnaround point, I found out why I didn't have much trouble in the first half of the ride. I had been pushed along by a fierce wind that was now like a cement wall I had to push through on the return trip. As I sat in my saddle acting like a sail catching the wind, I started to see the benefit of having tri-bars that would have reduced my wind resistance.

I was spent by the time I reached the transition zone, but had forgotten all about my full bladder as I started the run. Thank goodness the run was always the last event. It was my comfort zone, and I flew through the run to the finish line, even passing a few of the racers who had out-swum and out-cycled me. I finished in the top half of the competitors, making me start to think I could be good at this if I trained.

At the brunch and awards, Denard took first place, as predicted, in the over-forty category. I was in the top five of the thirty to thirty-nine group. But I noticed there was only one other competitor in Denard's category and if I were forty, as I would be next year, I would get a prize.

I could now legitimately claim that I had done triathlons. I had even exceeded the Olympic distance. But I couldn't let it stop at that. I felt like I belonged in triathlons and decided I would do more of them and look at even placing in the top three next year, once I was in the over-forty category.

Frank Dunn Triathlon

With three triathlons and several running races behind me, I was starting to feel much more like an athlete than a couch potato. I couldn't even recognize myself when I compared the image in the mirror to pictures from the past. I no longer craved beer, liquor, and cigarettes; I was now addicted to racing and I couldn't quit—nor did I want to.

I signed up for my fourth triathlon, which was to take place in Prince Albert National Park, the annual Frank Dunn Triathlon—1.5 km swim, 62 km bike, and 13 km run. It was also a Canadian Ironman qualifier, meaning that the first-place woman and man would receive a spot in the annual Penticton Ironman race, which was competitive to get into as it was a qualifier for the world championship race in Hawaii. I didn't care about the Ironman spot; I only wanted to race. I needed to race.

It was a hot day—over thirty Celsius by the time the run leg started—but I loved every minute of it. The water was colder than I had experienced, and I still didn't have a wetsuit, but it was the least intimidating swim I had seen yet as the route ran parallel to the shore, giving me a psychological boost. The bike ride was a wonderful scenic route through the national park, and even on my old bike, with the rack still on the back, I was able to pass some competitors. Another cyclist and I kept trading spots, he overtaking me on downhill and me him on the climbs. Even in the heat the run felt great and had become my favourite part of the race. I always overtook many runners, and this day even more runners than usual fell to my rear due to the heat, which didn't seem to affect me.

Again I felt that sensation as I crossed the finish line. This high lasted for hours after each race, and I always craved the next event. No prize for me in the thirty-to-thirty-nine group, and Murray and Denard took first and second in the over-forty category. It looked like there was a third spot waiting for me in the over-forty category for next year, and I planned on claiming it.

Having now competed in four triathlons and several running races, I was seeing the same faces over and over. I was becoming part of the circuit without even knowing it. I now had people to talk to and share stories of the race. I felt like this was my home.

Season 3

My off-season now had a purpose. I would be forty years old before the next race season began and I hoped to win some medals. If I picked the right races, I should be able to finish in the top three. However in the bigger races, my competitive category would still relegate me to the lower ranks.

Marlene had been very supportive of my transition over the past number of years and was my groupie at most of my local races. In recognition of and appreciation for my new obsession, she bought me a new bike for my upcoming triathlon season. Well she didn't actually buy the bike; she wouldn't have known what to look for. She gave me a birthday card with a picture of a bicycle and a directive to buy myself a new bike. I now wouldn't look so out of place in the hi-tech transition zones. As much as I would have loved to go right to the top of the scale of racing bikes, I knew our finances would only allow me an entry-level racing bike. I purchased a brand new Bianchi for about six hundred dollars, and I made sure I got the proper clipless pedals, the attachments to fit on the bottom of my used biking shoes, replacing the obsolete model from the draw prize I won in my first race.

I also made contact with the Regina Cycling Club and began joining in some of their club rides and weekly time trials. Triathletes were not considered real cyclists, so I never received a warm welcome, but I wasn't there to make friends, rather to improve my cycling skills. Through Sask Sport the club had the services of a full-time coach and manager, Warren, who went out of his way to help me improve my cycling skills. I was even invited to their winter training camp. I flew with the club to Las Vegas, where we and our bikes were packed into some vans and trailers and driven to the small town of Hurricane, Utah, to spend a week of cycling in and around Zion National Park.

I also kept up my regular swimming schedule at the Lawson Aquatic Centre during the off-season. My swimming style was improving, but my speed was only marginally better than the previous year. I was now bumping into more of my fellow athletes whenever I went for a run, swim, or a bike and was feeling more a part of the racing community.

I planned to do as much of the Timex Road Race Series as I could, and I hoped that I could take in all of the available Saskatchewan triathlons. Don and I did considerable running together, and as much as my speed was improving, his was improving at a much faster rate, due to diverting his attention from his crumbling marriage to his running. He was now much faster than I was.

Estevan 10K Race

Running your age—the magical goal of weekend runners. For most in their thirties, this was only a faint dream. But I was forty now. It should be possible—a forty-minute ten-kilometre race. My fastest to date was forty-two minutes, but this was a new season, the first race of the year, in Estevan.

I had been able to run under four minutes for one-kilometre intervals, but could I sustain it for ten full kilometres? I had been training with a heart rate monitor, so I was familiar with my limits.

Don and I traveled together to Estevan for the first race of the season. He and I had close times in all our previous races, but he had lost a lot of weight during a painful divorce, had used running as his escape from reality, and was in the best running condition of his life. I was sure he would beat the forty-minute barrier. But he was only thirty-six years old, so even if he beat forty minutes, he wouldn't run his age.

Estevan was a small race compared to others in the Saskatchewan Timex series. It only attracted about fifty runners, so I thought there was a good chance I could place in the top three in the masters category. I saw Tisdale runner Al at the start line, who was ten years my senior and a legend on the Saskatchewan running circuit. I had been in several races where he participated, but had never even been close to him. He didn't even know who I was. That's the way racing is; you only know the people in front of you, never those behind you.

Everyone sprinted off at the sound of the gun. Don was up with the leaders, and Al wasn't far behind. I pushed my heart rate to 172, knowing I could sustain that for long periods of time. I was able to keep Al in sight, but Don was way out in front, beyond my view.

By the five-kilometre mark I realized that I was not far behind Al and may even be gaining on him. At the turnaround point of the out and back race, I saw Don coming my way and he shouted, "Go get him! You're gaining on him!"

I saw that Don was having the race of his life, but I also was running my fastest race ever. I was 19:30 at the halfway mark. Forty minutes was possible if I could maintain this pace. I never let my heart rate fall below the 172 mark, but I also knew that I had some reserves, as I had trained as high as 177. At the nine-kilometre mark I decided to push to my maximum, knowing I could sustain that for the less than four minutes it would take me to finish.

Al's back was getting closer and I felt like Wile E. Coyote chasing the Roadrunner. With just over five hundred metres to go, I reached for all my reserves and blew past Al. He didn't know me, and it didn't seem to cause him any concern.

I crossed the finish line in 39:50—I did it, and I beat Al, who crossed about fifteen seconds after me. I turned and congratulated him and shook his hand after he slowed down. His first words to me weren't "Congratulations" or "Well done," they were "How old are you?" When I replied, "I'm forty," he scowled and pounded a clenched fist onto an imaginary table. "Damn!" he shouted. Never so much as "Good race." My image of a sportsmanlike older runner was shattered. He made me feel like I had robbed him of a treasure.

It turns out this was the first time Al had lost the Estevan masters division. I took first place. My first sub-forty time and my first win.

Don finished in a spectacular 37:24. Al never beat me again and never forgave me, nor would he give me the time of day. He now knew who I was.

Prince Albert—Longest Day Run

I was addicted. I had it bad. I needed a fix. I had to drive three hours from Regina to Prince Albert to get my next fix. The Prince Albert Road Runners club was holding their annual Longest Day Run at 8:00 p.m. on a Saturday night. If I left at 4:00 p.m., I could get there in time to register, relax for a while, and then warm up before the race started. It was the only way

I could get my high that weekend, and I needed it. The awards would be around 9:30 or 10:00 p.m, I could be back on the road before 11:00 p.m., and I would float home and hopefully be down from my high by 2:00 a.m. when I would be in bed.

I was pretty sure Al would be in the Prince Albert ten-kilometre race, as his hometown, Tisdale, was only a short drive from Prince Albert. I needed to know that my sub-forty-minute time was sustainable and not just a fluke. I also needed to know if I was now really faster than Al or not. My addiction and competitiveness were showing.

I arrived in Prince Albert just before 7:00 p.m. The prairie sun hung above the horizon to my left the whole trip. That time of year, the sun stayed visible until late in the evening. And as far north as Prince Albert, it didn't get dark until 11:30 p.m. That, of course, is why they call it the Longest Day Run. You could have a late evening event entirely in the daylight.

Prince Albert is not a large town, so with the directions from the registration confirmation I found the race site with little effort. I was one of the first to check in, but before long others started to line up to register. I ran across David, one of my running rivals from many races over the past couple of years. He was considerably slower than me in the races, but he always enjoyed the events. Being a similar age, we had hit it off and always hung out at the races. I knew he would be there, as this was his hometown.

"Hi, Brian," David said. "I want to introduce you to your competition. Brian, this is Rod. Rod, Brian Borgford. You two should have quite a race."

What was he talking about? I had never even heard of Rod. He never raced in any of my races. Al of Tisdale was my competition.

Regardless, Rod and I seemed to have a lot in common, and we ended up talking and comparing training and racing until the marshal announced that the race would begin shortly.

Rod, David, and I all shook hands, wishing each other a good race. Al was still not speaking to me after his previous loss, so we didn't connect before the race. He had the bug worse than I did.

The gun sounded and we were off. I set off at a fast pace, looking to finish my first kilometre in 3:45. I knew that the first kilometre was always my fastest, so I didn't want to start slow. Rod sprinted out in front and Al held back, but not too far behind. I knew he had me in his sights; he wanted revenge for the Estevan race. My heart rate monitor settled in at the one hundred seventy mark, so I knew I had reserves if I needed.

Rod set a good pace, so I just let him stay in front, but within reach. I didn't want to make a move too soon and expend my reserves motivating him to higher performance. Al seemed to fade farther back and I soon even forgot he was in the race.

At about the seven-kilometre mark I decided to push it. I bumped my heart rate to 175, knowing I had at least a couple more beats per minute if I needed them. Al faded farther back and I caught up to Rod, who wasn't that far ahead. I decided that I needed to put some distance on him to try to discourage or deflate him, so I pushed to 177 beats per minute and left Rod in the dust. I was at least five hundred metres in front of him and felt that I could easily keep him behind me for the rest of the race.

By now the younger fellows who were leading the race were out of sight. I was leading the next pack and was the leader of the masters racers. It's nice to be in front, but there is a risk and you need to know the route.

This was my first time in Prince Albert. I had committed the cardinal runner's sin of not properly studying the race route; I had not driven the route prior to the race. This was a normal ritual of mine, but I'd neglected it this time. The race marshals were usually parked strategically to keep you on course. Not this time.

I was well on my way to beating my forty-minute time, which was my primary focus now that I knew I had first place in my grasp. Al was a few hundred metres behind me, and Rod was now behind him. I felt comfortable and I felt fast. I rounded a corner and took a left turn. Al and three other racers followed me. The five of us galloped at full speed until we heard someone shout, "You're going the wrong way!"

I had led this little procession almost two hundred metres down the wrong path, and we all had to turn around and return to the proper race route. As I sprinted back to the corner where I had erred, I could hear Al utter some none too kind words indicating his extreme dissatisfaction with my sense of direction. Although the race marshals are there to help out on the race route, they are just volunteers, and it is the responsibility of the racer to familiarize himself with the route. I had failed to do that and had no one to blame but myself. Al obviously didn't share my sense of responsibility.

I watched with despair as I saw Rod make the correct turn and take a substantial lead. But I wasn't prepared to give up yet.

I poured on the coals and thought I could push extra hard to the end of the race. I knew my theoretical maximum heart rate was one hundred eighty beats per minute and I had never encroached on that territory until now. I pushed up to 179—a new high for me—but I was still alive, so I kept pushing.

I caught him. Rod and I were now running shoulder to shoulder. I was sure that I could push harder and leave him behind again. But the more I pushed, the more he matched me. The final five hundred metres were all downhill. I gave it all I had, while Rod and I kept pace with one another. I gasped for air but wasn't prepared to slow down. Then I made the mistake of looking at my heart rate monitor. I wished it had an off button; I would have turned it off right then. It read 186 beats per minute. Theoretically, I was dead. My heart was not supposed to operate above one hundred eighty beats per minute.

This slight hesitation gave Rod the opportunity he needed to pull ahead. Rod crossed the finish line in 38:46. I was a couple of strides behind at 38:52. I finished second, but I was elated. All I wanted to do was beat Al and beat forty minutes. I set a new personal best, taking second place, while Al finished third at 39:32, faster than my pace in my Estevan win the previous month.

Once we caught our breath, Rod and I congratulated each other. He too had set a personal record. My presence had spurred him on to greater effort than he had ever achieved. Al still refused to partake in postrace congratulations. He obviously blamed me for the error on the race route and wasn't speaking to me.

Rod was magnanimous in accepting his first-place prize. He attributed his win to my error, which caused him to be the accidental champion.

However, I had another theory. Had I not made the mistake on the route, I would likely have finished in a comfortable first place at about 39:30—probably just ahead of Al, who was gunning for me. Getting lost pushed me to even greater effort and gave me the ability to actually break thirty-nine minutes, which up until now didn't seem possible.

For me, second place was just fine. The personal record was more important to me on this special day.

Rod, David, and I sat together and compared race stories until it was time to pack it in. The sun had set, but it was still dusk when I hit the highway for the long return trip.

I had received my fix and I floated all the way back to Regina, not even noticing the remaining daylight dwindling off to my right. I think I still had a grin on my face when I woke up the next morning.

This high would last for another week before I started to crave my next fix. I knew I was badly addicted. But I didn't need rehab.

Disaster

The World Masters Games were coming to Regina in July 1992. I had never heard of these games before, but I found out that they included a series of physical, and not so physical, competitions for those who were too old to ever get a shot at the Olympics. Many of the events were copies of those held at the Olympics. They didn't have any middle-distance running events, like five- or ten-kilometre races, they only had short events such as one- and two-hundred-metre sprints. Triathlons were still under consideration for the real Olympics but hadn't filtered to the Masters Games yet. However, I did notice that they had two cycling events. One was a forty-kilometre time trial, which was a perfect fit with my triathlons and associated training. The other was a ninety-kilometre bike race. I decided to enter the time trial, but I had never even considered a bike race. In spite of my involvement with the Regina Cycling Club, which actively promoted bike races, I didn't really like riding in the packs, as it required so much concentration and discipline. If one person made a mistake, it could take down thirty other riders. But a couple of my triathlete buddies planned on entering the bike race as well, so I capitulated and entered both events.

The time trial took place on a typical windy day on the prairies and I didn't have my best time, finishing in about sixty-five minutes. Some of these world class cyclists, many of whom were ten to twenty years my senior, completed in some impressive times, the winner coming in at forty-eight minutes. I don't think I even made the top ten in my division.

The bike race was another story.

I wrote the following for a writing contest. It describes the tragic end to my debut season as a forty-year-old runner and triathlete. This event took place after I had already completed a duathlon in Moose Jaw, placing second behind Denard, and the Saskatoon Olympic distance triathlon, where I took third place behind Murray and Denard.

I see people through a haze. Slow motion, looking at me. I can't breathe. A man says to me, "Take your time. Breathe slow." He says something else that I can't understand. I gasp for air. I can breathe now.

Pop...sssss. A noise comes through the foggy air. I see a funny-shaped circle spewing an inverted cone of air.

I start to talk. I don't know why. "Yes, it's broken." I reach below my left shoulder and feel a bone pushing under my skin. I feel very calm, but confused. People are all around me. One young fellow sits on the ground and pushes his back against mine to keep me from moving.

"The ambulance is on the way!" someone shouts out. "Just keep him from moving!"

"Just keep still, help is on the way," a voice tells me.

Now small talk. Why do I have to deal with this?

"Great day for a race." "Good turnout." "Quite a crash." More disembodied voices.

What is all this nonsense? What am I doing here? Where am I? It looks like a highway. Why are all these people here? Why am I the centre of attention?

Little thoughts and memories start to form. The circular shape is a bicycle wheel—all bent up. Hissing air. Looks like my bike. It's not even close to me.

The guy pushing his back up against mine keeps talking. "How are you feeling?"

"I'm OK," I reply. "I think my collarbone is broken, but it doesn't hurt."

"Just hold on for a few more minutes, the ambulance is almost here."

"Let me wipe off some of the blood," said another voice. Blood? What blood? One fellow dabs above my eye. "Does that hurt?"

"No, not at all." I don't feel any pain, but I am not comfortable sitting on the highway with a fellow pushing at my back.

"It's here, clear the way."

What's here? Oh, the ambulance.

A giant in a uniform starts to examine me and asks a bunch of questions. He and a uniformed lady lay me on the road and check me out. Three people lift me carefully onto a wooden board. They strap something around my head and lace me tightly to the board. I can't move. They have fastened my head to the board and the pressure is pulling the hair on the back of my head. That hurts.

Up, floating. Onto a wheeled buggy and pushed into the ambulance. As the door closes one guy shouts at me, "That's the best crash I've ever seen! Three bounces!"

What about my car? What about my bike? Some things are coming back. My bike is lying on the road. My car is in a parking lot somewhere nearby.

"Don't worry, someone is taking care of that." Myron is the name on his nametag. (Myron, I remember meeting him many years ago. He got his girlfriend pregnant and as a fundamentalist Christian, he had sinned. He was devastated. Thank goodness for me, he got over it.)

"I'd better let my wife know. Is there any way to contact her?" I ask Myron.

"Sure, I have a cell phone here. What's the number? Her name? Hi, Marlene? My name is Myron. I'm an EMT and I have your husband here...No, he's OK. You can talk to him. Here, Brian."

"Hi there. I think I'm OK, so don't worry. I just wanted to let you know what's happening. Apparently they are taking me to the General Hospital. You can meet us there."

Lots of small talk. I think I remember what happened. It was a bike race. I remember starting the race. I remember the pack and trying to keep up. I don't remember it ending. I must have crashed. That's how my collarbone broke. But nothing hurts, except the darned back of my head where the hair is being pulled by the board I am strapped onto.

Here we are—straight to emergency. I'm still strapped so tight I can't move anything. Marlene meets me in the emergency room. Her face is white and she has a forced smile on her face. Oh, she has Tony, my son, with her.

"We are going to take a few x-rays," a nurse tells Marlene. "We'll only be a few minutes."

My favorite cycling jersey and they just sliced it in half with shears.

"Looks like nothing's broken other than the collarbone. You were lucky." A doctor looks at some black-and-white negatives with a bright light behind them.

Off come the collar and straps. Now I can move my head and stop the pain of my hair being pulled.

"But we need to tend to that gash above your eye." He brings out a long needle.

"What's that for?" I ask.

"Just a bit of freezing. You need a few stitches."

"Why not just go ahead and stitch? I don't feel any pain. I don't need freezing."

"Your choice. If you don't want it, I'll just stitch."

The needle feels strange, but it doesn't hurt.

Marlene and Tony come in. "Will he need an operation?" Marlene asks the doctor.

"No, we don't set collarbones. He'll just have to get used to the bone sticking out. It's not that far out. Just a sling will do it. Keep it immobile for a few weeks."

"Hi, Morley," I say as Morley enters the emergency room. "What are you doing here?"

"I just wanted to see how you were doing. I felt pretty bad about running over you."

"Running over me? When was that?"

"When you went down, I couldn't get around you and I rode right over your stomach."

"I never felt a thing. I must have been right out of it. Anyway, don't worry about it."

"Well, I hope you are back racing soon. Your front wheel is finished, but the frame should be OK. Your helmet is in pieces, I guess it did the job," he says as he leaves the emergency room.

"What happened?" Marlene asks, still looking very pale.

"I think I was on the third lap, about 60K in, when I must have crashed. I can't really remember. I was coming down the hill at about seventy klicks. I wanted to ditch a water bottle and that's the last I remember."

"Well, it looks like you won't be racing for a while."

"I'll probably miss the rest of the summer triathlons, but hopefully I'll be ready for the marathon in October."

Obviously I'm pretty lucky. This was my first real bike race. I jinxed it when I said good-bye to Marlene this morning: "See you later today, unless I crash."

I think I'll stick to running.

I had a full racing season planned but that was now over. I had preregistered for every race I could find. I had even put a deposit on a cabin in Prince Albert National Park for the Frank Dunn Triathlon in August. All for naught.

This was the year I was planning to strike the third item off my list—the marathon. Several Regina runners had planned to travel to Minneapolis for the Twin Cities Marathon in the fall. I was determined to be recovered for that race. Although I couldn't run for a long time yet, I could still get on the exercise bike after about a week of recovery, with my arm still in a sling.

Once I received assurances from the doctor that my collarbone, which was sticking out in a sharp point, was fused, I began to run. Slow, short distances at first, then longer runs, and finally back to some speed work. My addiction pulled at me more than my smoking and drinking ever did.

The Twin Cities Marathon

I managed to fit in enough training and fully recover in time to participate in the Twin Cities Marathon in October 1992. Marlene and I drove to Minneapolis and stayed with my brother and his wife who lived there. A good-sized contingent of my fellow Regina runners also drove down for the marathon. Not one of the bigger marathons, it still had about six thousand competitors, making this the largest race I had ever attended.

If it hadn't been for my bike crash, I had expected to do my first marathon in a time of three hours and ten minutes, perhaps even as fast as three hours. Now with the setback in training, I was hoping to make the Boston Marathon qualifying time of three hours and twenty minutes for my age category, forty to forty-five years.

We started at the Metrodome—or as it is often called, the Humphreydome—the Vikings' and Twins' domed stadium, named after former US vice president and Minnesota senator Hubert Humphrey. Being my first marathon, I was nervous but confident, unlike my other first races. I knew I could do this. However, the thousands of people amassing at the start line created an overwhelming scene. The starting chute had a self-seeding system whereby racers were to stand in the section designated with their estimated finish time. I dutifully placed myself between the markers labelled 3:15 and 3:30, but I may have been the only one who followed the rules. When I looked around I found that most of the runners in this section were wearing headphones attached to a Walkman or in some cases wearing funny costumes. I knew I was not in the section with serious runners. I ended up paying a price in time for following rules. I was a long way back in the pack of starters.

When the gun went off to start the race, I could barely hear it, I was so far back. The pack didn't even move. After about a minute the crowd crushing around me started to shuffle forward, then accelerate to a slow walk, then a faster walk. We had reached a slow trot by the time I actually crossed the official start line, over three minutes after the timer had started.

These were the days before "chip" timing, so I was three minutes behind before I even started. I had taped some benchmark times to my watch to help me pace my time during the race, but these times became irrelevant given the pace the crowd forced me to keep for the first several kilometres. My first mile, targeted at 7:30 on my pace list, came in at almost ten minutes. By the second mile I had passed enough people that I was at a running pace, but still not at what I hoped was my racing pace. I was almost getting nauseous watching the sea of colours moving like ocean swells. At one point the masses had to run through a long underpass. Everyone thought it would be a great idea to start shouting and let the noise reverberate in the tunnel. I thought my head would explode from the sound.

I was close to the five-mile mark before I could reach my full race pace, and I was exactly three minutes behind my target time. I remember hearing from experienced marathoners never to push too hard during the first half of a marathon no matter how good you feel, as the second half is a killer. With that advice stuck in my mind like a mantra, I held back while still trying to make up for my lost time, even though I felt I could pick up the pace if I wanted.

Marlene, my brother Del, and his wife Aggie had driven down with me to the race and showed up at various points along the route to cheer me on. This was a big event in Minneapolis and Saint Paul, where the race would end at the capitol building, attracting a large crowd of spectators along the route.

Other than the bike leg of my Regina Beach triathlon, I had never experienced the need for a toilet break during a race. But a marathon is a different kind of race, and at the halfway point I had to use one of the plentiful toilets to relieve myself. I selected one of the portable toilets that had obviously been used by someone more desperate than I was. I only had to urinate while the previous occupant must have had a bigger problem, as there were feces all over the interior of the fiberglass unit. He must have exploded when he entered; it was disgusting.

I was now into the second half of the event and still feeling good, so I tried to pick up the pace. In spite of how good I felt, the previous thirteen miles had taken a toll on my body and I couldn't go any faster, but at least I didn't feel the need to slow down. When I reached the twenty-one-mile marker, a man and a woman I had been following stopped and moved to an area just off the race route to meet a small delegation of people. The funny outfits they were wearing included a tuxedo-like set of running shorts, T-shirt, and white collar and cuffs for the gentleman and a white running outfit with a veil for the lady. It turns out they were a couple who had met through running and decided to marry while running, and the delegation they met up with was the preacher and witnesses for their wedding. The ceremony only lasted a couple of minutes and they were back in the race, finishing not far behind me, the groom carrying his bride over the finish line.

I had been told that many a marathon ends at the twenty-one-mile mark as people faded, so I did a quick status check and I still felt good. I was still a few minutes off my planned times, but couldn't seem to make my legs move any faster. I tried hard to pick up the pace in the last couple of miles, but I was maxed out. I crossed the finish line at three hours and twenty-three minutes, three minutes off my planned time and exactly the amount of time I had lost at the start. But I wasn't disappointed; this was still a good time for a first marathon. I felt great as I crossed the finish line, being met by Marlene, Del, and Aggie. Once I stopped running, however, my body seized up, the effects of forty-two kilometres, or twenty-six miles, becoming evident. I couldn't even lift my leg to climb the curb.

The next day Del and Aggie wanted us to see the Mall of America and I spent an agonizing day walking miles through this mall. Fortunately the runner's high was still with me and I was able to survive the ordeal. I didn't care; I had done it, and the last item on my list now had a checkmark.

Season 4—And Then the World...

My winters—or the off-season, as I was now calling it— took on a whole new meaning in my life. My every action and activity was directed at improving my athletic abil- ity, mainly through hard, structured training. I was also more aware of what foods would aid me in my preparation without becoming a fanatic about diet, only about the training.

Preparation for season four was now underway. I was fully recovered from my bike crash, with the only evidence being a sharp bone sticking out from my snapped collarbone. I had found recovery from the marathon more of a challenge than I had ever anticipated. I did lots of proper structured training based on research in preparing to run the marathon, but I hadn't done any research on how to recover from one. After a couple months of lower-level activity, my body said OK, you can train again.

I continued my winter training with the cycling club; we held weekly indoor rides at the Regina Field House track and had several other training activities. I went with the cycling club on another winter cycle training camp to Utah and continued to improve my cycling skills and strength. I joined a triathlon swim group with proper coaching and instruction on training for long-distance swimming. I still ran on my own or with a buddy, like Don. Don had now gotten his ten-kilometre time down to thirty-six minutes with the unwelcome assistance of marital difficulties and an impending divorce.

I started the racing season by going to Estevan to defend my title with a thirty-nine-minute time and Al somewhere behind, still cursing me. The day after the Estevan race, I competed in a duathlon, run-bike-run, near Lumsden and took first place in the masters category. Two first places in the same weekend. I went to Saskatoon for the Bridge City Triathlon, my third time there, and I beat Denard, finishing second to Murray, but by the thinnest of margins. He was in my sight.

Then there was an Olympic distance triathlon at Kenosee, in Moose Mountain Provincial Park. The Saskatchewan Triathlon Association billed this as their provincial championship event, which meant nothing to me—I just wanted to race. I finished first in my division, again beating Denard, but Murray did not participate. This race included an open water swim in what was usually the calm, shallow waters of Lake Kenosee. However, on this day there were gale force winds making the out and back swim a challenge, battling high waves and wind. I was officially labeled with a thirty-seven-minute 10K run, but it was obvious the distance was well short of ten kilometres.

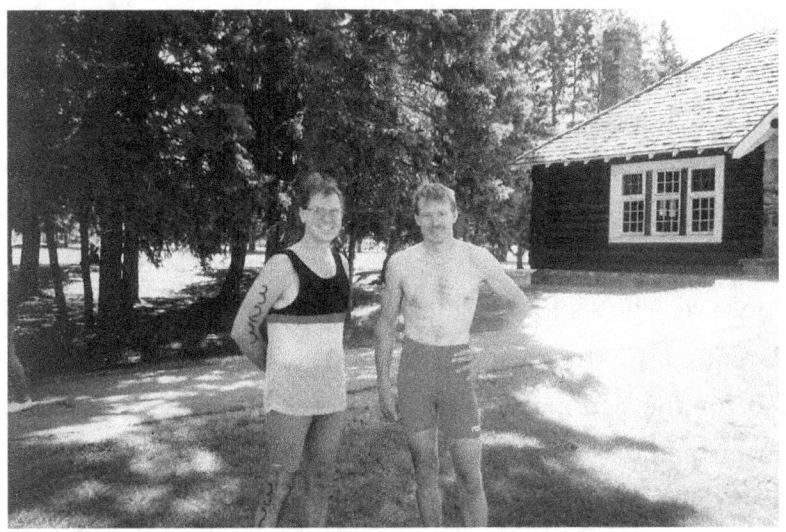

With Denard (on the right) after one of my early triathlons

The week following the Kenosee race I received a phone call from Hank, the president of the Saskatchewan Triathlon Association, telling me that I had won the provincial championship and was given a spot on the provincial team that was going to the national championships in Calgary in a few weeks. I was astounded and grabbed the chance to go as part of a team.

I went to Calgary to compete against the best triathletes in the country with little expectation other than to set a personal best. I did so with a time of two hours and fourteen minutes, including a ten-kilometre run where I finally broke the forty-minute mark in a triathlon. I finished seventh in my category and was happy with that placement given my newness to the sport and the fact that these weren't just weekend warriors like myself, many of these were serious athletes.

Only days after returning home from the nationals, I received another call from Hank. He told me that my performance had earned me a spot on the national team and asked if I would consider accompanying the national team to the world triathlon championships that were being held in Manchester, England, in August. I almost dropped the phone. I had heard that the top four in each category at the nationals would receive a spot on the national team, but I was seventh. Hank told me that everyone in front of me had already qualified for the national team in other races. I would be one of eleven people in the country in the forty-to-forty-four-year age group. I accepted and planned on going to the race of a lifetime. I couldn't believe how far I had come in such a short time. I thought I must be a real athlete now.

I finished off my local season with a triathlon in North Battleford, where I again took first place in my category and won the season points total for my age group, beating both

Murray and Denard, whom I had looked upon as idols only a short time earlier, although I had never actually beaten Murray in a race.

Now I was off for my first international event.

Manchester

Although I was part of a several hundred-person national team, I still had to foot the whole bill myself. That included the airfare, accommodation, team clothing, and meals. Triathlon Canada, the governing body for triathlons, did provide considerable discounts for most things, but it still cost a lot of money, which I was happy to pay to be part of this event.

I flew from Regina to Toronto where most of the team, those who took advantage of Triathlon Canada's discounts, were boarding a plane directly to Manchester. I never did get to meet any of my fellow triathletes at the airport or on the plane. It wasn't until we got to the airport in Manchester before any of the Team Canada organizers brought people together for common transport to the hotel. We arrived one week before the actual race to allow team members to get over jet lag, see the route, and do some last-minute training.

While waiting in the Toronto airport, I ran across a group of former co-workers from a previous part of my life. I used to travel, drink, and party with many of them, and it looked like they were still performing the same routine. They choked and laughed when I responded to their question, "Where are you going?" "You're going where?" one of them replied as he dropped his jaw in disbelief when I said I was going to compete in the world triathlon championship as part of the Canadian team. They knew I had changed my life with weight loss and exercise, but this turn of events was beyond their comprehension. I'm not sure they really believed me when we parted company.

Manchester was one of the cities bidding for the 2000 Olympics and had secured the world triathlon champion-ship to support their claim that they could host world-class sporting events. At the airport the Team Canada organizers gathered us together and amassed our luggage and bicycles for transport to the hotel in downtown Manchester. We had a double-decker bus allocated to the team members arriving on this plane, and there was a lorry (truck for Canadian read-ers) to carry our luggage and bikes. En route I started to get a feel for Manchester and its reputation as an industrial centre. It seemed like a dirty, polluted, and crowded city not worthy of world-class athletics. Even the people seemed to be pasty white and sickly looking, probably from breathing the nasty air. *Good luck with the Olympic bid*, I thought as I watched the unattractive scene unfold on our way to the former cotton mill that served as our hotel.

The stone building didn't look like a hotel, based on my North American hotel experiences. The small lobby and tiny two-person elevator were not equipped to handle the hun-dred and fifty triathletes who descended on them this dreary August day, each with luggage and a bicycle. The elevator only held two people and one bike at a time if everyone held their breath; this was going to be a long day. Even with the team organizers taking the lead on registration, it took over an hour for us to get our room allocations and keys. I was on the third floor and waited my turn to get my stuff in the elevator to reach my room. That was the last time I entered the elevator. With a hundred and fifty people needing to get up and down several times each day for the week we would be there, the stairs made more sense, even with the bike on my back. Most people held a similar opinion; after all, we were athletes.

I still had not actually met any of my fellow competitors, so I was pretty much on my own. There were three others on the team from Saskatchewan whom I knew from racing and training. There were several triathletes from the Saskatchewan team who'd qualified for the national team but were unable to attend. Dave and Newel were two young fellows in the twenty-five to twenty-nine year category, and Fionna was in the elite (professional) category. I had been in many races with these three and all of us had attended the winter cycle training camp in Utah. Most of the team focused on the race and had little time for visiting and making new friends.

Once in my room, my first task was to get my bike together. I had disassembled it and placed it in a cardboard bike box, further making me look like a rookie compared to the custom-made hard-sided boxes containing all the hi-tech bikes. My new Bianchi, slightly dented on the crossbar from my crash, was still pale in comparison to my teammates' bicycles. I put everything together so it looked like it fit. This was the first time I had ever taken my bike apart and the first time I had ever put it back together.

I decided to have a short nap and noticed that there was still light coming in through the small window of my tiny but serviceable room. As I pulled back the curtain to the window, I discovered a brick wall with a tasteful florescent light at the top, giving the illusion of being a window. I found the switch and turned it off to have my snooze.

The team manager had given us a full schedule of events leading up to the race and our departure. We started out with a team meeting where the manager told us all the rules and regulations. I was taken aback when he talked about performance-enhancing drugs and potential random drug tests on the athletes. I was still just a weekend warrior and didn't know this was even an issue with triathletes, but in addition to us age-groupers, the race was for professional athletes.

We made several scheduled trips to the race site to scope out the swim course and some of the bike route. Most of the bike portion would take place on a freeway that would be shut down on race day. We couldn't see any of the running routes, as the run would take place in downtown Manchester on cordoned-off streets and at that time the downtown streets were a mass of vehicles and pollution. The swim was in a quarry near the town of Bolton, the bike leg was from Bolton to Manchester, and the run would take place in Manchester. This required two transition zones; one from the swim to the bike and one from the bike to the run. That added to the complexity of an already confusing event; I had barely competed in a half dozen races and could hardly be considered experienced. I was still discovering something new in every race.

Double-decker buses transported us from the hotel to the racing venues, and our bikes were loaded onto lorries for those who wanted to do some rides prior to the race. I only did this once, as it was a hassle to carry my bike up and down the stairs at the hotel. Also I was embarrassed every time the workers assigned to loading and unloading the bikes commented on how heavy my bike was compared to the others. I also found that waiting on the street for the busses to arrive gave me a headache. The pollution in the city was overwhelming.

On the various bus rides out to the venue and training places, I did get a chance to meet a few of my teammates, but everyone was so focused on the race that making new friendships was a low priority. I met two other professional accountants, one from Vancouver in the fifty to fifty-four category and one from Winnipeg in the thirty to thirty-nine category. The most interesting person I met was a gentleman from Northern Ontario by the name of Kurt. He was seventy-two years old and had been racing all his life. He was in the sparsely populated seventy-plus category. I thought he must be the oldest person in the race, or at least on the Canadian team, but there was one older fellow I never got to meet, though I followed his progress. Roman was a seventy-nine-year-old racer from Montreal and the oldest person in the race.

Kurt had the misfortune on one of his training rides to be hit by one of the double-decker buses, probably with the confusion of having to ride on the opposite side of the very narrow roads. Although he was messed up a bit, he didn't have anything more than some bumps and bruises. It would slow him down in the race, but not eliminate him.

The day before the race we had to set up our two transition stations and make sure they had everything we would need for race day, as you wouldn't see them again until the race. I had already been in one race with two transition zones, but they were within walking distance of each other and that was before I had to worry about separate shoes for the bike and the run. In this race the transition zones were over forty kilometres apart. Supposedly your items from the first transition zone would be transported to the finish area after everyone was out biking and they would be waiting for you at the end of the race.

I mentally rehearsed every step I would have to take before and during the race to try to remember what to put where. I was now a faithful wetsuit user, so I would have to bring my wetsuit with me on race morning. I had a couple practice swims in the quarry near Bolton and was happy to have the wetsuit. The water was cold, no colder than what I had experienced in Canada this summer, but cold enough to make you appreciate the protection the wetsuit provided. The racers from the warmer climates, like the South Africans and Australians, found the entire venue of the cold, wet English summer difficult to adjust to.

I would have to have my bike, helmet, and biking shoes at the first transition, but I would also need to leave my bicycle pump there, as the tires always needed a top-up before a race. Due to the cold weather and the luxury of using the wetsuit, I would be able to dress completely for the bike before the race, wearing my cycling jersey and long Lycra pants with Canada written down the legs under my wetsuit. At the first transition, I would drop off my wetsuit, don my helmet and shoes, and be off. Oh yes, I would also leave some warm clothes in the transition zone for transport to the finish line. I would be damp at the end of the race and would appreciate the warmth.

The second transition zone would be slightly easier. I would only need my running shoes and a hat, which I always wore when racing. Here I would park my bike, doff my helmet and cycling shoes, put on my hat and running shoes, and head out on the double loop of downtown Manchester and cross the finish line. Then I would retrieve my warm clothes, which would be waiting for me, and head off to the postrace festivities. I was pretty sure I had it all figured out and carefully put my things in my prenumbered transition stations. I was a bit leery of leaving my bike, as I had never before arrived on race day without it, but all fifteen hundred competitors had the same issue.

I was now as ready as I possibly could be.

Late in the day before the race, all teams were required to participate in the opening ceremonies on the grounds of the city hall in the town of Bolton. Each team was required to wear their team uniforms and march in as a unit in a predetermined order. The Americans were the largest contingent, looking smart in the flag colours. The Australian team was the second biggest, with their dark outfits and a broad-brimmed hat to match. Everyone envied their uniforms, especially the hats. The New Zealand team made the biggest splash. The forty to fifty competitors also had dashing outfits. They stopped in the middle of the procession and started to chant and stomp in a Maori war chant, a *haka*. Everyone watched in fascination as they spent about five minutes chanting and dancing, making a dash to the steps of city hall to conclude their performance. They received an ovation from the large local crowd that had come to watch the procession in support of the race and to hopefully support the bid for the Olympics.

The Canadian team looked presentable, all in our red outfits with no headgear.

We were large, but didn't stand out. We assembled at the end of the ceremonies for a group photo on the steps of city hall where the Kiwis had performed.

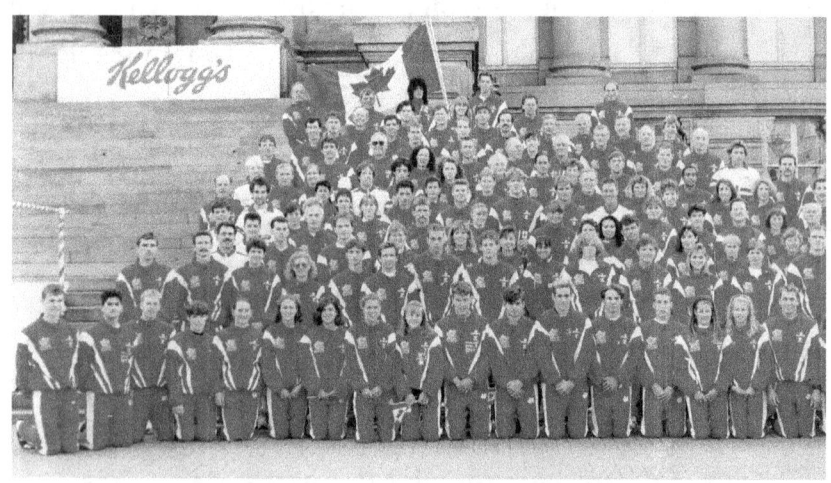

Team Canada in Manchester – 1993

(I'm in the second row from the top with the flag pole protruding from my left ear.)

Some of the smaller teams received huge ovations for their efforts, which must have been intimidating in the face of so many larger teams. The team from Iceland consisted of one lone athlete.

The ceremonies, complete with speeches from local officials and politicians, ended early in the evening and we were returned to our hotel to rest up for the race, which would start first thing the next morning.

Manchester Race Day

I was nervously confident on the bus ride out to the race start. I was amazed at how the polluted air had turned fresh for race morning. Downtown Manchester had been closed to all traffic for the race, resulting in an absence of fresh exhaust clogging your lungs. The constant mist and rain had also contributed to cleaning the air. The race venue, at the quarry in Bolton, appeared picturesque and serene as the hundreds of competitors began amassing to check out their transition areas. The overcast sky with light drizzle squeezing from the low clouds provided a postcard view of the green English countryside, complete with old stone fences and sheep grazing on lush pastures.

The swim would start in waves of about one hundred swimmers per batch. The oldest categories would go first, followed by each consecutively younger category, and finally the elites, or professionals. This order was used to provide as much concurrent activity on the route as possible for the thousands of spectators who had begun assembling along the forty-kilometre cycling route. This schedule would also provide the shortest gap possible between the first finisher and the last, creating excitement at the finish line.

We had to walk to the swim start area, which was in a different location than the swim finish. The swim was in the form of a V and would not require any repeated laps. It was well marked with buoys and ropes all along, so there would be no confusion on the route. There was between a hundred and hundred and fifty in my wave start. Although there was the usual mass confusion I had experienced in other beach-start open water swims, this was actually more orderly than I had expected. Some kicking and elbows, but I never felt intimidated, and within a hundred metres the pack was spread out enough to have a comfortable swim. I finished in a respectable twenty-six and a half minutes. I had hoped to do twenty-five minutes as I had done in a race in Weyburn earlier in the year, but at least I was in the middle of the pack, not near the end.

I whipped off my wetsuit as I sprinted for the transitions zone, and now I was ready to settle into what I expected to be an enjoyable but wet bike ride; it was still drizzling as I started out.

The first ten kilometres were on some beautiful narrow and winding English country roads. The curves and twists made for a slower pace than I had hoped for. We had been warned about one steep descent with a hairpin turn at the bottom. Apparently this road had been used in many movies with car chases in rural England. Given my experience from the previous year, I feathered my brakes all the way down the hill, refusing to let loose like others appeared to be doing. As I reached the hairpin turn, I was grateful for my caution, as I saw several racers ride off the road and into the ditch at the bottom trying to make the turn. Many of them got hurt or damaged their bikes, ending their race at that point.

After the picturesque part of the ride, we entered a free-way called the M-something. It had been completely closed to all vehicle traffic, giving us the whole road to maneuver. Thousands of people cheered along the route. I often heard "Go, Canada!" in a thick English accent as people saw my team colours and the word *Canada* printed down the side of my long cycling tights.

We had been told of a long uphill climb once we were on the freeway, and they were right. It was over five kilometres of steady climbing—not like climbing the mountains in Utah, but enough to force me into my lower gears for longer than normal. I survived and cruised into downtown Manchester to the second transition zone. My speedometer read forty-six kilometres, not the forty as billed, not that it mattered as we all had to ride the same distance. The extra distance and complex route had given me a much longer bike time than I expected, close to seventy-five minutes.

With fifteen hundred transition stations, it took me a while to find my spot, even after rehearsing my location the previous day. I parked my bike, doffed my helmet and cycling shoes, slapped on my Brooks Kona racing flats with the Velcro closing tabs, and sprinted out of the transition as fresh as if the race had just started. This was always my favourite part of every race.

I felt like I was floating with effortless leg movement. I'm sure the crowd's cheering helped push me on in the now clean air of Manchester with no traffic to clog the lungs. I couldn't figure out the route, but it really didn't matter; the route was lined with a metal fence to keep the spectators from interfering with the runners. All I had to do was stay between the fences and with the growing pack of runners. It was a double loop, and I couldn't tell one loop from the other. I was passing runners, runners were passing me; I couldn't tell whether I was gaining or losing, but I felt great. As I saw the finish chute ahead of me, I could hear someone panting behind me. I didn't want to be passed by anyone in the last couple hundred metres, so I pushed to the maximum. I didn't wear my heart rate monitor in triathlons, so I didn't know what my heart rate was, and I didn't care. I just wanted to keep this guy behind me. I crossed the finish line with a run time of 39:20, my fastest ten-kilometre time in a triathlon. Checking the results afterward, the guy breathing down my neck was an Irish fellow in my age category who had just run a thirty-six-minute ten kilometres; in spite of his superior run time, I was able to fend him off at the finish.

My overall time was two hours and twenty-six minutes, nowhere near my better times, in spite of my excellent swim and record run. The extra distance on the bike and the large, confusing transition zones had contributed to a slower overall time, but I would have to wait and see how I fared against all the other competitors when the results were posted.

Feeling my usual elation at the end of a race, I looked for someone to share my experience with. But there was no one. Dave and Newell, my Saskatchewan buddies, were still on the racecourse, having started in a wave well behind me as they were in one of the youngest categories. The elites had not completed yet, but I saw Fionna's husband who informed me that an aggravation of an existing injury had put her out of the race.

I looked for the usual snacks and drinks that normally were shoved at you at the end of a race, but there was nothing. I was now getting chilled in the cool, wet English air and began looking for the van with my gear and warm clothing that was to be transported from the first transition zone. It had not arrived yet and no one seemed to know when it would come. The disorganization and lack of support at the end of the race started to erode my runner's high more quickly than usual. Feeling a touch dejected after the race of my life, I decided to walk over to my hotel, which fortunately was near the finish line. Other teams were not necessarily as lucky with their locations. The hotel had the European method of dropping your key at the desk every time you went out, so I knew I could get into my room. In other circumstances, my hotel key would be in the gear that had not arrived yet.

When I got to the hotel, there was a crowd gathered on the street and the hotel was filled with police and firefighters. There had been a fire alarm and the hotel had been evacuated.

I couldn't get to my room and still had to stand in my wet, sweaty racing clothes in the cloudy Manchester drizzle. No one had any idea when this emergency would end, but it was becoming clear it was a false alarm and the officials took their time to clean up the loose ends. I went back to the finish line to await the arrival of the transition truck. It took over an hour for it to finally arrive, and I was relieved to be able to pick up my gear and cover with some warmer clothes. I carried my bag of stuff, retrieved my bike, and walked back to the hotel, which was now operating as normal. It was great to get showered and into some clean, warm clothes, but I still hadn't been able to share my experience with anyone—and that was half the fun of racing.

I finally got to meet up with some of my teammates and share stories from the race that evening at the awards ceremonies and social. I found that one of the traditions of the world championships was to trade uniforms with triathletes from other countries. Although our uniforms weren't as attractive as some, I was still proud to possess the many pieces I had earned—a warm-up suit, Lycra cycling pants, singlet, sweatshirt, swim trunks. I did capitulate to some extent, trading a couple items for some South African cycling pants and an Australian running singlet.

I pored over the results when they were distributed. Out of fifteen hundred racers, I was about eight hundredth, just below the middle of the pack. Sounds like a low finish, but I was in the older groups of racers, and this race included the best triathletes in the world, not just some weekend warriors.

In my category I was ninth out of eleven Canadians, not near the top, but it told me I was in the top ten in Canada and that made me feel good. I was fiftieth out of seventy-five entries in my category, near the bottom, but the bottom of the best in the world.

Kurt, the seventy-two-year-old I had met, was only about fifteen minutes behind me and took the silver in his category—the seventy-year-plus category. Roman, the seventy-nine-year-old and the oldest person in the race, had finished near the end of the pack, but was far from last. I competed in another race he was in two years later. He was eighty-one then and still not last. Dave and Newell were in the top thirty of their category, and although Fionna had to pull out, her friend Joanne Ritchie, from Kelowna, took third place in the professional category. The previous year, Joanne had been the fastest woman and Fionna seventh.

I got a brief chance to meet one of the Canadians in my category who had beaten me and taken first place at the nationals in Calgary the previous month. He was racing with his family, and although none of them won any prizes, his wife finished in the forty to forty-four women's category, his son in the twenty to twenty-four category, and his daughter in the under-twenty category. Impressive: four from the same family qualifying for the team and competing at the worlds. Dave Dawson of British Columbia placed seventh in my category with a breathtaking time of two hours and five minutes.

The following day most of the team was shuttled off to the Manchester airport where our plane was delayed by five hours.

I had a tight connection in Toronto, so I knew I wouldn't make my flight to Regina. Once we did finally get into the air, the pilot acknowledged the Canadian team on board and congratulated Kurt for taking the silver in his event.

The plane made up almost all of the time we had lost in the delay and we touched down with lots of time for me to catch my connection—that is if the customs officials would have worked a bit faster. They wouldn't fast-track me to make my flight and Air Canada would not hold my flight for even a few minutes to let me board. I arrived at my gate for the flight to Regina just as they had closed the door to the airplane, and they wouldn't reopen it for me. Although they put me up at no charge in the plush airport hotel, I really wanted to get home to share my experience with my family. From the time I crossed the finish line in Manchester, my positive experience was filled with little glitches. But even those glitches couldn't erase the fact that I had gone from a fat couch potato to a world competitor.

Life After the Worlds

That was twenty years ago, and I have been training and racing ever since.

My original motivation, to display a life of health and fitness, was to set a better example for my sons, who were young when I embarked on this journey. So I insert this section to show how my efforts came full circle. I am pleased that both my sons embraced health and fitness as a life priority so that they may too set a good example for their children. I would like to think that my example helped set the stage for their views on fitness. My younger son, who later became addicted to running, and I ran together often, and one time we even entered a ten-kilometre race together, he in his twenties and I in my forties. He was able to finish within thirty seconds of my time.

Years later, Cam trained hard, while I ran with him whenever possible, so he could compete in his first half marathon. I decided to be his main cheering section rather than compete in the race. I beamed with pride as he crossed the finish line in a time of ninety-six minutes. He was now in his mid-thirties, a similar age to when I started running.

Cam's Half Marathon

Standing at the start of a race with hundreds of people around me ready to try for a personal best, I felt strangely out of place. Of the dozens and dozens of races I had attended, this was the first time I had ever stood near the start line in jeans and a shirt rather than shorts and a running top. This wasn't my race. It belonged to my son, Cam, who was running his first half marathon. I couldn't be more proud as I watched him mull around the crowd of fit runners in his T-shirt, shorts, and ball cap, taking off for short jogs, followed by some light stretching in order to warm up.

The journey to this race could be viewed as a three-hour drive from Calgary to Edmonton, but really it started twenty-five years earlier in Regina, where I made the decision to change my lifestyle for the sake of my young sons so they could see their father engaged in productive, rather than destructive, activities.

Although it took several years for this modeled behaviour to manifest itself in my sons, Cam did take up running in his early twenties. While we were roommates in downtown Calgary, Cam and I would go on training runs a couple times each week. At first I could beat him with ease on any of our various runs, especially during our hill repeats. But as time wore on, he could keep up with no difficulty and was now blowing me away on the hill runs.

We entered the Forzani's Mother's Day run, a ten-kilometre race, to test out the results of our training in race conditions. I took off like a shot at the sound of the starter's horn, leaving Cam looking around for me as he started off at a slower pace. If it weren't for that jackrabbit start, I might not have beaten him by the thirty seconds that separated us at the finish line, both of us finishing close to the forty-five-minute mark.

I had the good fortune to be offered exciting overseas employment opportunities in China and the Middle East, so running together was limited to the few times we could fit it in during my summers back in Canada. Cam was now married and had started a family, and although it was difficult for him to keep at the running, it was still an important part of his life.

With the demands of career and family, he found running to be a way to keep his mental and physical states intact.

In the spring of 2010, Cam called me from Canada to tell me of a race weekend his company was sponsoring that summer. He wanted to enter the half marathon and wondered if I would like to do it with him, or perhaps do the ten-kilometre event. I decided that I would just focus on triathlons for the summer; this race, which I would attend as a spectator, would be his and his alone.

When I returned to Canada for my summer vacation, I stayed with Cam and his family. Because his job allowed him to work from his home, we were able to run together almost every day. He was specifically getting ready for the race later in the summer, so I shared with him as much as I could about training for the race. Now I could only keep up with him when we ran at a recreational pace. His abilities exceeded mine, so I could only counsel him on speed work rather than show him. Although I was still a good runner, a sixty-year-old runner is not as fast as a thirty-five-year-old runner. I bought him a Garmin GPS training watch to help him measure and improve his performance. He was running with strength and comfort, so the only unknown for him would be how long he would take to run the race, not whether or not he could do it.

We made it a family weekend, Cam and Carrie, plus Rochelle (my second wife; Marlene and I had divorced some years earlier) and me. The only missing element was the children, whom we left with their grandmother, my first wife,

Marlene. The company-sponsored event was first class all the way, including hotel rooms as part of the race package for employees and their families. There was a runner's market, prerace meals, and goodie bags.

Race morning we arrived early at the venue to see all the preparations taking place. It was one of the best mornings you could ever ask for in a race—cool air and clear blue skies. Cam looked nervous but excited as he joined the crowd in the starting chute. My camera clicked, catching all the activity from a vantage point I had never seen before. I snapped one final shot as the gun sounded to signal the racers to get started—only a shuffle at first, given the crowds. But with the current chip technology, racers were no longer penalized for lining up far back from the start line—your race only began when you crossed the starting mat.

I paced around the start-finish area for the ninety-plus minutes I estimated it would take Cam to complete the out and back route. Rochelle and Carrie sat in the stands waiting for the finish while I found a place along the fence to watch Cam complete the final couple hundred metres, my camera ready to start the video of his completion.

I recognized Cam the instant he came into the grounds where the finish line was located. He looked strong and fresh and was beaming from ear to ear. I started the camera rolling and cheered, calling his name as he crossed the finish line. My wife still gets chills listening to my voice shouting, "Wait to go, Cam!" as he ran by my vantage point. Ninety-six min-utes, the official time, a four-and-a-half-minute-per-kilometre pace for the entire twenty-one-plus-kilometre distance. The Garmin trainer results showed a consistent pace and heart rate throughout, except for the sprint at the end, when the cheering crowd urged him on.

I could almost feel the runner's high myself as I watched Cam prance to meet up with us after he claimed his finisher's medal. I took more photographs to record this epic event. I was proud of my son, and I was proud of the fact that my choices from years earlier had had a positive impact on his life.

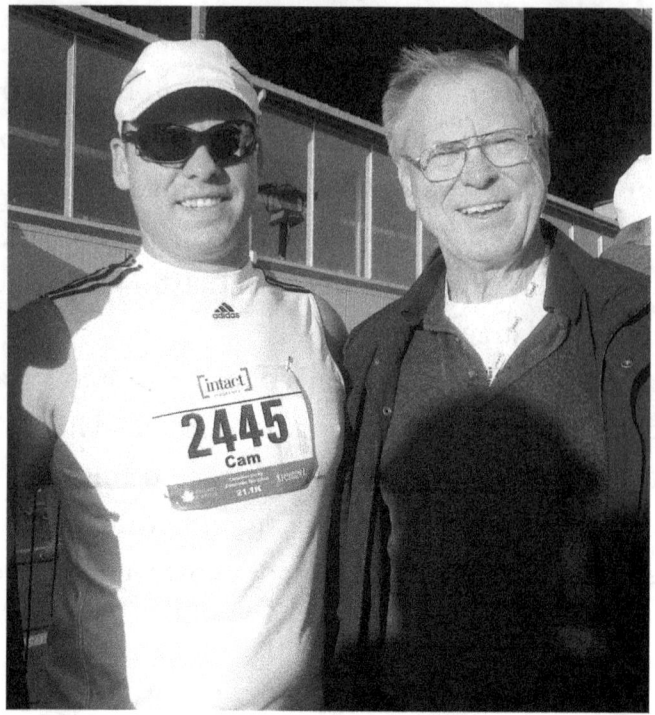

After Cam's half marathon

Encouraging Others

I made it my unofficial mandate to get as many people active in running and physical activity as possible. I was instrumental in getting my best friend, Chris, hooked on running and racing when he had said he couldn't see the point in it. He started running on my urging, just as a stress reliever for some turbulent times he was going through. Before long he was running races and training for his first marathon. He competed three times in the Victoria Marathon.

Chris unfortunately died of cancer far too young. Ironically, I married his widow several years after divorcing my first wife. I ended up putting together a marathon-training plan for her daughter, Lori, who wanted to compete in the Victoria Marathon, Chris' favorite race, as a tribute to her late father. I trained with her as much as possible, especially on her long runs, which she found difficult to get motivated for. She was elated to finish the race comfortably. I competed in the half-marathon event in that race and was there at the finish line to cheer her on. She gave me a big hug as thanks for helping her accomplish this tribute to her father.

I lived in Yellowknife for a few years and continued my training and racing there. I ran year round, including in temperatures as low as minus forty-six degrees Celsius. I ran in many communities across the Arctic, including Baffin Island and on the Beaufort Sea. Running in the winter in the Arctic can be quite a challenge, not only due to the frigid temperature and usual high winds, but because there is often little or no daylight. I was always a curiosity to the Inuit people of these communities who couldn't understand why this *kabluna*, or white man, would engage in such a stupid activity.

While in Yellowknife I competed in and organized many races, including running races, duathlons, and triathlons. I even raced on New Year's Day in minus forty temperatures. I helped organize a Learn to Run group where I saw overweight and out-of-shape women go from not being able to walk a block to running five kilometres straight. For many of them it was a life-changing experience.

I organized weekly bicycle time trials for the many cycling enthusiasts I met in this Arctic city. The local newspaper, always hungry for items, often sought me out to contribute to their sports section. I kept them supplied with articles, race events, and results.

I also lived in China for a year. I was unable to compete in any races, as I couldn't find any in the northeastern province of Liaoning. However, I was able to get some of the college students I was teaching off their backsides and out running with me. Some of them are running to this day.

I moved to the Middle East near Dubai for several years and dominated the fifty-year-old category in the many races they held each year. I learned how to run in extreme heat and humidity. Many of my training runs were in temperatures of forty-six degrees Celsius and above, and some of the races were in temperatures above thirty-five degrees.

When I turned fifty-five and fell into a new age category, I wanted to test how I would fare in heavy competition. So I ordered a new bike—a Cervelo, my first real triathlon bike—so I could spend the summer racing in Canada, where I travelled for summer holidays while living in the Middle East. I registered for six races that summer, almost one every week.

My first race of the year was in Edmonton and was a qualifier for the national team. I knew I couldn't make it to the world championships due to work commitments, but I wanted to see if I still had it in me to qualify. I arrived in Calgary after a thirty-hour flight on a Thursday night. The next morning I went to the cycle shop where I had ordered my new bike by e-mail from Bow Cycle and picked it up. I had never even seen it before that day, let alone ridden on it. I also purchased a new wetsuit, helmet, shoes, and all the accessories necessary to race. On Saturday morning, I borrowed my son's car and drove up to Edmonton for the race, which would take place on Sunday. Being a qualifying race, it was a structured event requiring racers to set up their transition zone the night before. It was cold and raining in Edmonton that weekend, a real shock after leaving the heat of the desert only a couple days earlier.

Still jet lagged and using a new bike that I had never ridden in weather that was outside my comfort zone, I hoped for the best. Because I had no chance to ride the bike ahead of time, I needed some minor tuning from the mechanics on duty immediately before the race. I swam a twenty-five-minute, fifteen-hundred-metre time for the swim leg—my fastest since I was forty years old—I had a respectable bike time for an unfamiliar bike on an unfamiliar route, and I ran the ten kilometres in forty-six minutes for a total time of two hours and thirty-two minutes. That was good enough for third place and good enough to qualify for a spot on the national team had I so chosen, but I declined the offer. I'm sure I could have finished under two hours and thirty minutes and moved into second place if I had been better prepared.

I won every race that had a fifty-five category that summer. I even won some that only had an over-fifty category, and I never finished below second place in my category. I still had it in me.

Not wanting to transport my bike back and forth across the globe, I purchased a Scott Plasma triathlon bike to use in the Middle East. I now owned two hi-tech racing bikes, a far cry from my old beat-up bike with the carrier on the back I had used in my first year of racing.

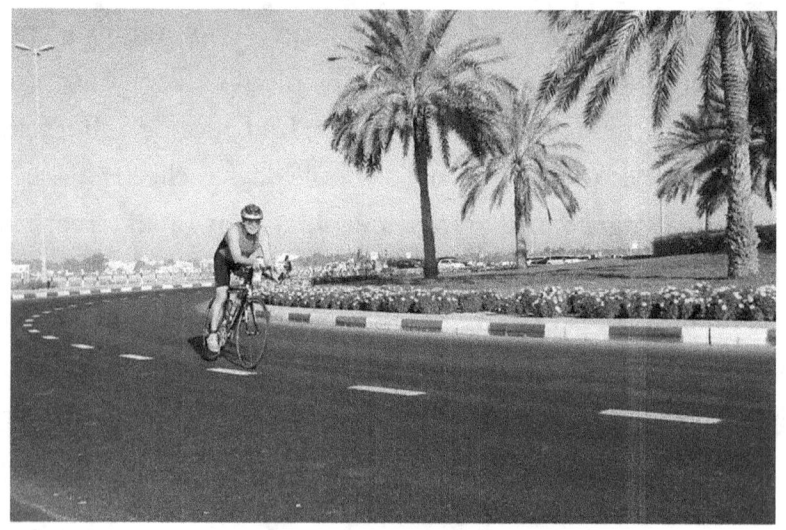

On my new Scott Plasma

As a fifty-nine-year-old in one Dubai race, I was able to finish an Olympic distance triathlon in less than two hours and thirty minutes, proving to myself that I wasn't slowing much. As a sixty-year-old living in Doha, Qatar, I was usually the oldest competitor in any of the various races sponsored there and still managed to be very competitive, even finishing second overall in a mini-triathlon at Qatar University, making all the young Arab boys competing wonder who this old guy was who kicked their butts.

I always think of the man I saw racing into his eighties. I hope that will be me some day. So if this story inspires you to start down a similar path, you can wave to me as I breeze by you in your first races. I'll be the old guy on the hi-tech bike.

Training

The following section outlines some of the training activities I have seen and participated in. It is not meant to be prescriptive, but rather to give some idea of how others get fit, stay fit, and train for races.

Learn to Run Program

With very few exceptions, anyone can run. That doesn't mean everyone wants or needs to run, but don't use the excuse "I can't run." People complain about knees, ankles, and other ailments from running. These are just symptoms of taking the wrong approach to running, usually running too hard or too fast when your body isn't ready for it. Often people, when starting to run, do a three- to five-kilometre run on their first time out and feel great. So the next day they do it again, then again. This is an aggressive approach that is destined to failure and probably injury.

If you want to run, you need to take a deliberate and gradual approach to embarking on a running lifestyle. Years of enjoyable running lie ahead when you tackle it sensibly.

Earlier I talked about helping organize a Learn to Run program in Yellowknife. The group was sponsored by Body Works and the owner/manager, Terry Chang. We started with about twenty-five participants, mainly women, as men don't seem to think they need any outside help with athletics. The few males who joined failed to follow the discipline, opting instead to show their machismo. We lost most of them either to ego or injury. The women all succeeded in the program and the results were staggering, both physically and mentally. These were changed people at the end of the ten-week program.

We started with the assumption that all the participants were healthy enough to make this journey, while encouraging them to get clearance from their doctors. Although healthy, most of them were far from fit, mostly overweight, and many of them morbidly obese. But they were determined.

The program was based on twice-weekly workouts with the group and one or two individual workouts. We suggested a maximum of four outings each week to allow the body sufficient time to rest and heal. Each outing was one hour, including warm-up and cooldown. We started embarrassingly simple and easy, increasing the physical activity gradually each week for ten weeks.

The first night out we started with a good stretching session, to warm the muscles and work on flexibility. Most novices have tight, contracted muscles, so they can't afford to take an aggressive approach or they will damage the muscles. Just light stretching, with no bouncing. You can find a stretching routine in any fitness magazine, book, or website.

Then we hit the road. The workout was broken into five-minute intervals. We separated into groups of five to eight runners, with a leader in each group who carried a whistle. We started by walking for four and one half minutes, at which point the leader would blow the whistle and everyone would run at a slow, comfortable pace until the leader signaled the end of thirty seconds with another blow of the whistle. We'd carry on in this manner for just over thirty minutes and would then do a cooldown, with more stretching. This stretching was a bit more aggressive, as the muscles were now completely warmed up and malleable enough to handle longer stretches.

On to week two, where we would do exactly the same routine, but now the walking interval was four minutes and the running interval was one minute. The third week we added thirty more seconds to the run and deducted thirty seconds from the walk. By the second to last week, the run was now four and one-half minutes and the walk only thirty seconds. Most participants shuddered at what they knew was coming in the final week—running twenty minutes with no walking breaks. But they all did it. They all graduated from the Learn to Run program and were now declared to be runners. Almost all continued their running after the program was finished. By the end of the official program you could see the physical changes taking place in the ladies. It was easy to spot the graduates' happy and proud dispositions when they realized they were now runners. In the months that followed the official program, some of these ladies underwent profound physical transformations. One obese lady lost over eighty pounds, became physically attractive, and was courted by a prominent lawyer in town, eventually becoming a couple.

I have shown this program to many others since then to encourage people into a physically active life. Once you have completed working through this program you can consider yourself a real runner. Then it is just a matter of running regularly, and you can participate in five- and ten-kilometre races. When racing, if you want to improve your times, you can start on structured training programs that will make you faster. Most people are happy just to participate.

If you want to move to longer distance racing, you need to get a little more serious about how you prepare.

Marathon Training

Anyone who runs can do a marathon. But it would be unwise to attempt one without proper preparation. To run a comfortable marathon that you can walk away from takes considerable time and dedication. So if you want to do your first marathon, be prepared to give up much of your free time for several months prior to the race. You should not attempt your first marathon without starting from a solid base of running, probably a year of regularly running five to ten kilometres three to four times per week. There are stories and even movies about people who crawl across the finish line. Some races will actually disqualify you if you are not upright when crossing the finish line. This is to discourage people from putting their lives at risk doing races without proper preparation. All races require you to sign a waiver stating that you have properly prepared for the race and you absolve the organizers of any responsibility. Your objective should be to cross the finish line erect, still running, and with a smile on your face. That makes you a winner.

If you decide to run your first marathon, you should develop a training plan that works for you. Searching the Internet or a bookstore will give you a plethora of ideas to build your plan. Jeff Galloway is probably the foremost authority on marathon running, especially for first-timers. His most recent Galloway Method starts from the premise that anyone can run one mile. And if you can run one mile once, you can run one mile twice. He suggests that you break your first marathon into twenty-six one-mile intervals, separated by short breaks. You won't set any records with this method, however many runners have logged some impressive times using it. The main objective is to get people to finish their marathon.

I'm still of the old school that believes you should run the entire race non-stop, but that's just a personal preference. I have developed my own training plan based on extensive reading about different methods. Mine is no better or worse than anyone else's plan, and like all the other plans, it works. I have proven it over and over again. I have used it in my own marathon training. I trained my ex-wife (even after she was my ex-wife, but that's another story) and some of her friends to success-fully finish the Yellowknife and Victoria Marathons, and I also trained my wife's daughter to complete her first marathon. All ran across the finish line with big smiles on their faces.

My plan incorporates several components, all of which should be used throughout the training to ensure a safe and comfortable race, injury-free. You don't need to follow it religiously, and if your body needs a rest at any point, listen and take a break. I generally recommend that each workout, except the LSD (long slow distance), be at least sixty minutes long, including warm-up and cooldown.

The components:

1) Long slow distance (LSD). This is probably the most important component to any marathon-training pro-gram. Unfortunately for many first timers, this is the only component in their training plan. To finish a mar-athon comfortably, you need to incorporate the other training activities as well. The distance you run on any given LSD outing will vary, starting with as little as ten kilometres and gradually building to forty kilometres four weeks before your race. The LSD should start with some light stretching, and then move to a very slow run, "embarrassingly slow" was what one running expert wrote. These should be done once every week, increasing by one or two to four kilometres each week until you reach the forty-kilometre level. Some advo-cates suggest doing your long runs every two weeks, but I prefer to see one every week.

2) Speed work. This can be unstructured (fartlek) or structured and is designed to help you improve your speed. I prefer structured workouts, but you select yours based on your personality. During the speed portion of the workout you should run at full capacity, far faster than you would ever run in any race. You maintain that level for anywhere between one and four minutes, depending how far you are into your marathon training. You need to run slow or walk for a couple of minutes between each sprint.

3) Tempo runs. If possible you can incorporate five- or ten-kilometre races as your tempo runs. A tempo run is running between 90 to 110 percent of your race capacity. This allows your body to handle the stress of a faster pace for extended periods of time. The fast part of the tempo run should last at least twenty minutes, with a proper warm-up and cooldown at the start and end.

4) Hill training. This builds your power and strength. Find a hill that is steep enough to make you work, not just a gentle slope. The hill should be long enough that it takes you at least ninety seconds to run up. After the appropriate warm-up, you run the hill at a comfortable pace and then walk or slow jog down. Then you turn around and do it again, only this time harder, completing it in less time than the first one. In the early stages of your training, three repeats are sufficient, but you want to build up to five to six repeats. Finish with an appropriate cooldown.

5) Cross training. This will allow you to maintain your fitness without adding to the stress on your body the volume of running is causing. Cross training could be cycling, swimming, stair climbing, elliptical training, or any other aerobic activity.

6) Warm-up. This is essential to avoid injury during your training. The LSD incorporates its own warm-up, so use this for all the other activities. Start with a five- to ten-minute light run. Then stop and do five to ten minutes of long slow stretching. There are many stretching routines you can follow, but make sure you work on the big leg muscles and your back. Stretching is meant to increase your flexibility. Never stretch cold muscles and go easy on the stretching after your body is stressed from long or intense activities.

7) Cooldown. This is designed to bring your body from the stressed state of a workout back to normal (whatever that is for you). Try another five to ten minutes of slow running, followed by five to ten minutes of light stretching.

8) Weight training. This is a useful component to build overall body strength, as you have primarily been working your lower body. Hit the gym two to three times each week but only for thirty to forty minutes. Remember you are training for a marathon, not the Mr. or Ms. World competition. That being said, upper

body and core body strength is imperative to successful running.

9) Rest. This is probably most important component after the LSD. You are putting considerable stress on your body with this training plan and your body needs time to recover. Build in one day each week where you do absolutely nothing physical. This is a good time for sitting on the couch watching movies. If your body starts to feel fatigued, don't be afraid to take two days off in a week, just don't do it every week.

I take each of these components and map them onto a schedule with the seven days in the week over the twenty weeks leading up to the marathon. With this map, you can then check off each of the components as you do them every week to monitor your progress. It is not essential to complete 100 percent of the items, but if you fall below 80 percent, you are starting to jeopardize your success. I have attached a sample training plan to show how you might build your own schedule.

Triathlon Training

For my first two years of triathlons I took a random approach to triathlon training, and then as I looked for dramatic improvements I turned to a more structured approach. One book I found particularly useful was Rob Sleamaker's *Serious Training for Serious Athletes*. It is not intended for the novice racer, but there are lots of tips that can be used by anyone.

The one measure that still sticks in my mind from reading that book so many years ago is that ten hours of training per week will place you in the top 10 percent of your category in your country. The simple message is you get out what you put in. Once I started getting serious about my racing, I always targeted ten hours of training per week. In recent years, I don't always reach that level, but it's still my target. Whether I'm racing or not, my ten hours of training produces positive returns. Even now, in my sixties, my daily productivity is more than the average person.

I was a self-taught swimmer, and my first couple of racing seasons produced surprisingly good results. Going into my third season, I got proper coaching, which made a world of difference, not just to my swim times but my comfort and confidence in the swim leg of every race.

Every child learns to ride a bike, so when you become an adult it is easy to take it up again. But I wanted to do more than just ride a bike, I wanted to race. The professional coaching I received from the Regina Cycling Club was invaluable.

I never did get professional coaching for my running, but I associated with many excellent runners and learned what I could from them.

After you have tested the waters, so to speak, with triathlons, you may want to seek out professional help—no, not a psychiatrist, although people have said...

I am not a coach nor an expert on any of these events, but I have years of experience behind me. I can't tell you what will work for you; I can only show you what worked for me, and still works for me.

The Swim

As mentioned, I am a self-taught swimmer. When I was young, I would go to the neighbourhood swimming pool with my buddies to splash around and jump in the water. All my friends wanted to go to the deep end, but you needed to prove to the lifeguard (my favourite was Pigeon, a cutie in a two-piece swimsuit) that you could swim two widths of the pool or you were banned to the shallow end with all the toddlers. I worked and worked at it until I could go across and back without going under.

We had a swimming pool attached to the high school I attended, and in phys ed class we spent some time learning various swim strokes. I adapted very well, learning all the strokes, but I really only enjoyed the freestyle, or the front crawl. Everything else seemed like too much work, especially the butterfly.

One summer I swam across a small lake in the Okanagan Valley, just to prove to myself I could do it. When I entered university, we had a compulsory swim class where I enrolled at the intermediate level as I was not a beginner and I didn't want to put in the effort that would be required in the senior level. In our first class, I had to rescue a classmate who was bubbling around in the deep tank on the directions of the instructor. He thought he was in the pre-beginner class and dutifully followed the instructor's directions, almost causing himself to drown.

Swimming is all technique. A certain level of fitness helps, but I have seen people far less fit than I beat the trunks off me in a swim race. While racing triathlons in Dubai, I always beat one of the competitors in my age group, Frank. Frank was a short, portly fellow, fifty-five years of age, same as me at the time. Depending on the distances, I would zoom by him on the bike or glide by on the run while he was obviously struggling. But I had to wonder why I always had to pass him to win. I was a good enough swimmer that I thought I should have been ahead of him in every leg, but he was out of the water minutes before I was. I finally asked him how he became such a good swimmer, and he replied that he was a former member of the US Olympic swim team. So even though I was in far superior physical condition, his swim technique never left him, and he was still one of the first ones out of the water, even as one of the oldest racers.

I joined a triathlon swim group in my first couple years of triathlons in order to work on my technique. It did make me faster and more comfortable in the water. While in Yellowknife, I joined a masters swim club and continued to work on my stroke. For me the secret was long, full strokes, not too deep in the water, and keeping my body straight and my legs near the surface. For triathlons, kicking was not as relevant as the arm stroke.

If you can't swim, you can't do a triathlon. If you swam as a child, you can likely pick it up again. If you have never swum, I can't help you. Considering myself a reasonably good swimmer, I have tried to coach friends in swimming and have learned that I am a swimmer, not a coach. There are ways of learning to swim later in life, but I have no clue how to get you there. So my advice to non-swimmers is to find some good lessons if you want to do triathlons,

I try to swim at least twice each week, although three times is better. I currently work at a college with a twenty-five-metre pool, so I can swim five days per week. I try to make sure I swim at least fifteen hundred metres each time, but if I'm able, I move it up to two thousand metres. I am usually in a twenty-five-metre pool, so I break my workouts into ten-lap segments, or two hundred fifty metres.

My first ten laps is a warm-up, consisting of alternating between the crawl and breaststroke. I then do ten laps with a kickboard, doing two laps of the flutter kick associated with the crawl and then two laps of scissor kick from the breast-stroke. My next ten laps use a one-armed drill to work on my technique—fifty metres with my right arm and fifty metres with my left arm. If I am on a training day working on drills, I move to breathing drills. I start with one lap breathing every fourth stroke then one lap breathing every fifth stroke and so on until I reach every eight strokes. Then I decline each lap down to breathing every fourth stroke again.

Most of the rest of the workout is devoted to speed while making sure that my stroke remains as close to perfect as I can make it. My target pace for a race is twenty-five minutes for fifteen hundred metres, so I use that pace as a target for my speed workouts. I try to do my one-hundred-metre intervals under one minute and forty seconds and in my faster sprints aim for one minute and thirty seconds. I also do longer intervals of two hundred fifty and five hundred metres, still trying to maintain or beat my target race pace. I finish up with a ten-lap cooldown of easy crawl and breaststroke.

Although I have only reached my target of twenty-five minutes twice in all my races, once when I was forty and once when I was fifty-five, I am usually under twenty-seven minutes. I still believe I will see twenty-five minutes again.

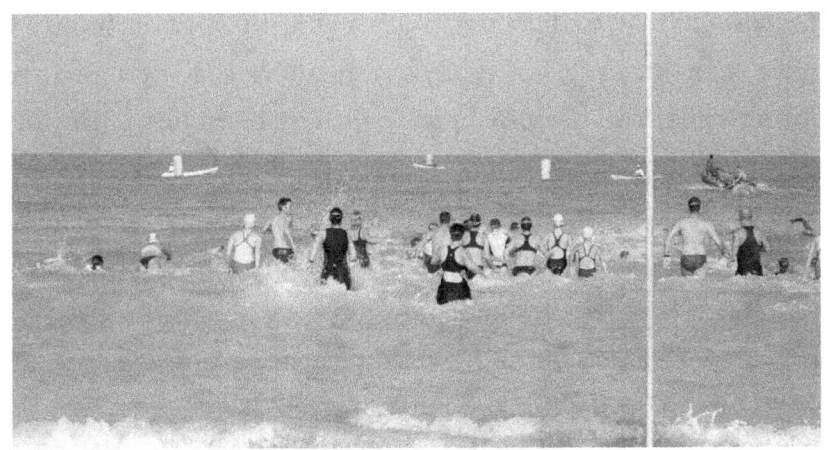

The start of an open water swim

The Bike

My dad bought me my first bicycle when I was seven years old, and he ran alongside me, holding onto my seat until I could go on my own. I have been on a bicycle most of my life ever since. My first bike was a CCM with coaster brakes. As I approached my teens, I graduated to a three-speed with a Sturmey-Archer shifting mechanism. By age fifteen I was going on weekend camping trips with my buddies with our camping gear strapped to racks on the back of our bicycles. Our trips were as long as one hundred miles. So when I started into triathlons, the distance was never a problem, I just needed to work on speed and power.

Although not to the same extent as swimming, cycling is mainly technique. To cycle well, you need a good level of fitness, but to cycle fast, technique seems to win over fitness. I have been out-cycled by many short, fat cyclists, often British. John Williams, a British brass polisher (his job was to polish the brass railings at the Hotel Saskatchewan), was several inches shorter than I, ten years older, and had a middle-aged paunch. I came within seconds of beating him in our forty-kilometre time trials, but I never did beat him. One short, pudgy real estate salesman in Regina also beat me every time, and I was in far better shape than he was.

Having a high-quality bike makes some difference, but the engine that powers it is the key. Once you reach your peak with whatever equipment you use, you can then consider moving to a better bike. Until then, it will make you look good in the transition zone but foolish on the course.

Cadence is the key to cycling. You want to maintain a cadence of eighty to ninety rpms (revolutions per minute) with your pedals. That is why racing bicycles have so many gears—to maintain cadence in all terrains. When I was young, a ten-speed was the bike of choice. Now I ride a racing bike with twenty gears. Each gear is only a small increment bigger or smaller than the previous in order for you to shift gears as often as necessary to maintain your cadence.

Your speed is impaired by two factors: wind resistance and rolling resistance. To minimize wind resistance you want to make sure you have tight-fitting clothing. Flapping fabric slows you down. A sleek bike with bladed spokes helps, but crouching down low, keeping as much of your body as sleek as possible, is more important. This is why triathletes and time-triallers use aero bars on their bikes; it keeps them out of the wind. Rolling resistance is caused by extra weight and wheels that don't rotate smoothly. You can try to make your bike as light as possible, but the weight of the rider is more important. Lose the flab. The more you train, the more this takes care of itself.

I try to cycle two to three times per week. More would be better, but it is often difficult to get to a good cycling route that is free enough of traffic to feel safe. While living near Dubai, I would go out one day on the weekend for a casual ride with some friends, a forty-kilometre route we would do in about ninety minutes. I would then do one ride on my own on a flat, straight road, trying to reach my race pace. I target a forty-kilo-metre-per-hour average, but as I get older that is getting harder to achieve. I often settle for a thirty- to thirty-five-kilometre-per-hour pace. In my forties, I came close to reaching the one-hour mark for the forty-kilometre distances but never broke it. Now in my sixties, I am happy if I can break seventy minutes.

Hill work is an important part of bike training. I lived in the city of Al Ain in the United Arab Emirates, near a small mountain, Jebel Hafeet, that rose to twelve hundred metres above the desert floor over a ten-kilometre road, an average slope of 12 percent. Quite a climb. A fellow triathlete and I would climb that hill every week. We would cycle to the hotel near the top, in a time of fifty to fifty-five minutes, and drop off our bikes with my wife, who drove up in the car. Then we'd run the remaining three kilometres to the summit. This was a great "brick" workout (bike, run).

Whenever possible I try to incorporate speed work in my cycle training. This might involve going full speed for three to four minutes each interval with a rest in between. High-cadence cycling also helps improve the smoothness of your technique. I try to use a lower gear and hit rpms of 110 or greater for a minute or two at a time.

I have lived in places where it is very inconvenient to do outdoor training on the bike. This could be for traffic reasons or weather. In that case I train indoors, either using a bike trainer on which I can place my own bike or in a gym where the hi-tech stationary bikes are a good surrogate.

Most cycle purists insist on going for three-hour to six-hour rides regularly. If you are training for Ironman, the long rides are essential. As most of my races are seldom longer than forty to sixty kilometres, I seem to be fine with bike training of sixty to ninety minutes.

The Run

I swam and biked recreationally as a youngster, but I never ran unless it was from bullies. In high school phys ed class we had some sessions on running, mainly a mile run. The class was broken into groups based on speed. There was the six-minute mile group, the seven-minute mile group, and the eight-minute mile group. Although I was a skinny young lad, I was placed in the group with the fat kids, called the also-ran group. This just wasn't my sport.

I was coerced into joining the football team, as our new high school didn't have enough students to hold competitive tryouts. I was put on the team as a back-up right guard, a benchwarmer. On occasion I was put into play when the outcome of the game was already determined. When the quarterback called running plays requiring the guards to pull, he always pulled to the left, knowing I wouldn't be able to run fast enough to block for the ball carrier.

So I was just as shocked as everyone else when I became a runner and running became my strength, especially in triathlons. When I realized that I was actually pretty good at running and had a chance of winning some medals, I read and researched everything I could about running. My bible for the first few years was a green paperback book by Bob Glover called *The Runner's Handbook*. I read it from cover to cover and reread and reread pages that helped me improve my running and provided motivation and inspiration. For a while I subscribed to *Runner's World* magazine, and I still occasionally pick up copies from the newsstand along with *Triathlete* magazine. They are a good source of training tips and motivation. What I realized was that after reading about twelve issues, everything started to repeat. There are only so many ways to run hills or do speed work, and stories like mine became a dime a dozen.

Through all this reading and research, I developed my own approach to training, which follows closely what I outlined in the marathon-training plans above. I do long, slow runs, interval work, hill work, and tempo runs.

When training for triathlons, I try to ensure that I run at least four times each week and that each run has a purpose. My LSD runs tend to only be ten to fifteen kilometres long, unless I am specifically training for a marathon or half marathon. My tempo runs are usually the middle five kilometres of a ten-kilometre run. For speed work I use a heart rate monitor and increase the intensity with each interval, usually holding it for a minute or two. My middle interval, of six intervals, is the most intense, with my heart rate approaching my calculated maximum before using my last couple of intervals to bring the heart rate down.

For hill work I try to find a hill that will take me two to three minutes to run up at a comfortable pace. In the town where I lived in the Middle East there was a perfect hill near our home. After a warm-up I would run the hill in about two and a half minutes and then jog slowly down. My second interval would be about ten seconds faster. I would do a total of five or six intervals, with my second to last one being the fastest and the final an easy one. Then I would do a ten- to fifteen-minute cooldown run.

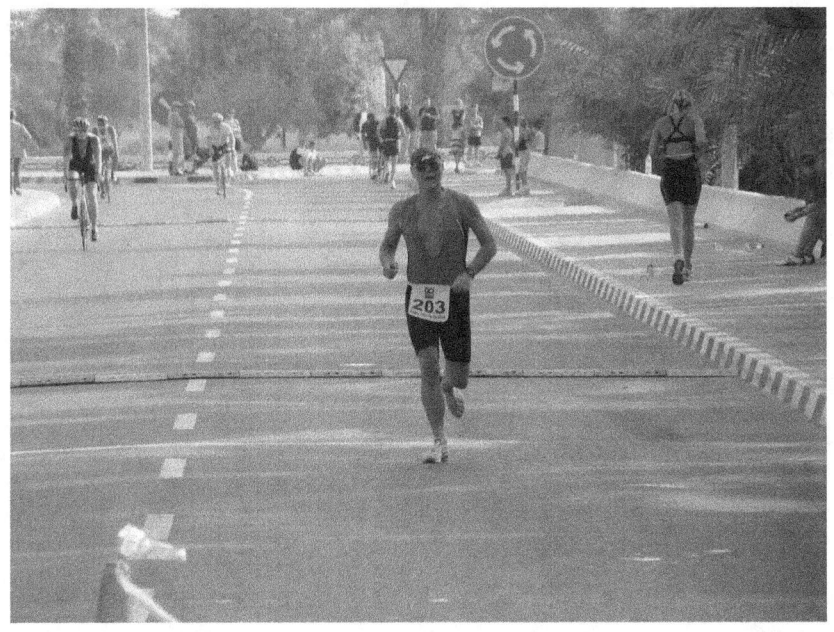

Near the end of a race

Odds and Ends

Clothing

The most important piece of clothing is your running shoes. Every name-brand running shoe company comes out with new and expensive gimmicks and features every year. These wonderful must-have features mysteriously disappear in time for the next model year. Since modern-day running shoes replaced the old gym sneakers starting with the running craze of the seventies and eighties, nothing new and revolutionary has really appeared. I always go with a name-brand runner (make sure they are running shoes and not for some other purpose), but purchase their least expensive low-end model. If there is a great sale on, I will buy two or three pair and put the extras in my closet for future use. I try to have two pair of runners on the go at any one time; I will discard one pair each year and replace it with a new pair, as the cushioning will go before the runner ever collapses. I place my discarded runners beside a dumpster in a neighbourhood where I know there are homeless or needy people, and they disappear fast.

For running, most T-shirts and shorts are fine, and unless I'm racing I wear ordinary white sports socks. In races, especially triathlons, I go barefoot to save time in transitions and just deal with the sores and blisters that may occur.

Newbies to triathlons can get by using their running shoes on the bike, but most people migrate quickly to clipless pedals and rigid cycling shoes that are more efficient at transferring your leg power to the pedals.

For cycling, tight-fitting clothing is best to avoid loose clothing flapping in the wind and slowing you down. Cycling shorts with a chamois or other padding in the crotch is almost essential. Cycling jerseys are expensive, but they last forever. I'm still wearing the cycling jersey that I crashed in many years ago. They had to cut it off me at the hospital, but I gave it to my mother-in-law and she stitched it back together like new.

In triathlons I wear a trisuit, which is a one-piece outfit with shirt and pants combined. When swimming with a wetsuit, I just pull the wetsuit over top. When I'm not using a wetsuit, a trisuit is great to swim in, and you don't need to put anything else over top when you exit the water. Race rules usually state that men must have their torsos covered. The same rule doesn't exist for women, but I have not seen women violating that regulation.

Marathons

Many marathons take place in the spring or fall as the summer heat can be a problem. As a result, the weather will vary during the marathon itself, cooler at the beginning and warming up as the race progresses. You will often see people dressed in warm clothing, gloves, hats, and jackets at the start of the race but only wearing a T-shirt and shorts at the end. Most races have drop-off points where you can discard clothing as you get too warm, and the organizers bring it to the finish line for collection later.

When running a marathon, it is almost impossible to avoid the peril of chafing or black toe, or with men, bleeding nipples. You can try various methods to avoid or minimize these hazards, but I consider it the price you have to pay for the feeling of success when crossing the finish line. These sores all heal while recovering from the race.

When running in winter climates, I add layers of clothing as the temperatures drop. While running in the Arctic, I would have as many as four layers of clothing, with the outer layer being nylon (many prefer Gore-Tex) to allow the moisture to exit the layers. At the end of my Arctic runs I looked like an icicle. Covering your head in cold weather is the most important consideration, as that is where you will lose much of your body heat.

Equipment

Other than running shoes and clothing, most of your equipment needs will revolve around your bicycle. However you should have a pair of swim goggles that fit firmly and don't permit leakage. I have tried all shapes and forms of goggles, and for me and the shape of my face, I always end up with the cheapest model with a neoprene seal. I have tried the expensive models, but they always seem to leak, and you don't want your eyes exposed to saltwater in ocean swims or the chlorine from pools. During one race in Weyburn, Saskatchewan, where I first hit the twenty-five-minute mark, my goggles leaked the whole race and one eye was full of green algae from the prairie slough were we swam.

As mentioned, most people move to proper cycling shoes as their first upgrade. The next item with the biggest payback is tri-bars. No other single piece of equipment provides a faster payback in time. My times improved by five minutes when I put a set of clip-ons on my first real racing bike. My next upgrade was to have the shifters put on the end of the tri-bars so I wouldn't have to get out of the racing position to change gears.

Bikes are all equipped with water bottle cages, or at least a place to install cages, on the down tubes of the bike. This requires that you come out of your racing position to drink water, and you will need water in your races. This is another time-waster in a race. Speedy drinking systems have come and gone with various degrees of success or failure. When I first started racing, many triathletes had a vinyl bladder affixed under their saddle with a thin hose leading to a spout at the handlebars, so a rider only had to bite the end of the hose and water would squirt from the pressurized bladder. This only lasted a couple of seasons and the pressurized bladders had a tendency to explode in the transition zone, leaving the rider waterless during the ride.

Most people with tri-bars now use a plastic bottle, available in most bike stores, that fits in the tri-bars and has a plastic straw that is close to your mouth when you're in the racing position. I have been using such a bottle for many years, and it serves the purpose. There is usually enough water to last me the forty kilometres of a triathlon bike leg, but I keep an extra bottle or two in my cages, just in case. For longer races, you can carry extra water in bottles in cages behind your seat.

Heart rate monitors are a great way to improve your training. As you can see from some of my races, they can be useful during a race to assist in carrying out your race strategy. While doing serious training, I have always used a heart rate monitor; Polar is the most common brand name. In recent years, I have moved up the technology scale and started using the Garmin trainers that work with a GPS system and heart rate combined. These are useful and fun, but not necessary, gadgets.

Many people like to train while listening to music on iPods or MP3 players (gone are the days of the Walkman). When training or racing outdoors, I find this to be an unnecessary and dangerous distraction. Many races now ban the use of music players during the race for safety reasons.

Swimming in Cold Water

Triathlons have rules as to when wetsuits are allowed, required, and banned. Above a certain temperature they are not allowed—about twenty-two or twenty-three degrees Celsius. Below a certain temperature, they are required—about eighteen degrees Celsius. In between those two temperatures, it is optional. Like most triathletes, I will wear a wetsuit whenever I'm allowed. First, it provides for mental security, knowing that you will not find it too cold during the swim. The second reason is that a wetsuit makes most swimmers faster. The buoyancy and sleekness lets you glide through the water faster than without the wetsuit. The better swimmers, those with a real swimming background, prefer to go without a wetsuit as their technique makes them just as fast with or without it. For me, my times are usually two minutes faster with a wetsuit. In races where wetsuits are not allowed, either due to water temperature or because it is an indoor swim, I have often shaved my legs, as excessive hair does slow your swim.

One mid-June race in Saskatoon, race organizers decided to use the South Saskatchewan River for their spring race rather than the usual venue of an indoor pool. Analysis of previous years made them believe that the water temperature would be high enough to have a wetsuit-optional swim and by this late in the season spring runoff would not be an issue. This turned out to not be a normal year. Winter was late in leaving, meaning that spring was late in arriving, as was the spring runoff. The water temperature was so low that wetsuits were compulsory; the water was high and flowing fast with the late spring runoff. The water was so cold that, even with wetsuits, several swimmers had to be hauled out of the water with hypothermia. This was the last race that I used a short-sleeved wetsuit; I could hardly feel my bare arms and shoulders during the swim, and the water, filled with debris, pushed me so hard I couldn't make the turn to the swim exit, requiring me to run several hundred metres extra to the transition zone. The good thing about the conditions was that the fast-flowing water gave me a swim time of nineteen minutes for what was actually eighteen hundred metres. The feeling came back to my arms and shoulders during the bike portion, but I couldn't feel my toes until about the eight-kilometre mark of the run.

The following year, the organizers opted instead for a shallow lake outside of the city, and conditions were more normal. The swim was wetsuit-optional, but they probably didn't check the water temperature. Due to the unnecessary use of the wetsuit, I overheated during the swim and felt faint and weak by the time I started the bike portion.

These two races are examples of the extremes you might face when racing. Most races have more predictable and less extreme weather.

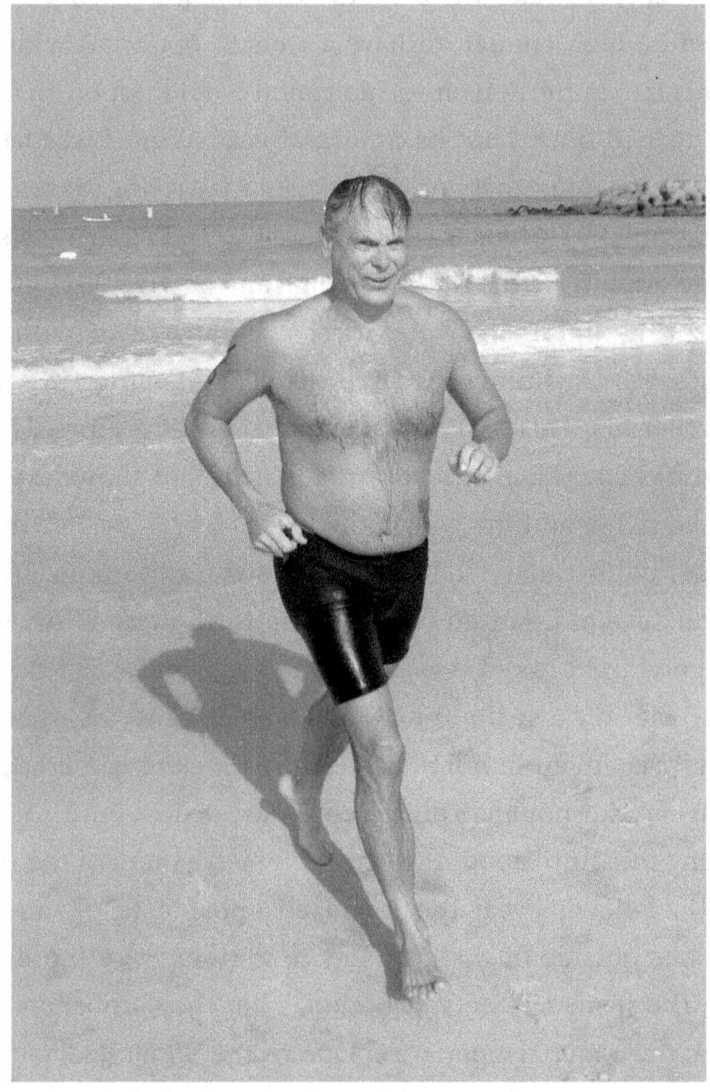

Exiting a sea swim

Running in Odd Weather

I probably made more trips to Saskatoon for races than any other city. They always seemed to be hosting running races or triathlons. One of their premier events was the annual marathon held on the last weekend of summer, the Labour Day weekend. This event consisted of the full marathon, a half marathon and a four-person marathon relay. I assembled a team of co-workers and we entered the corporate category of the relay, and I concurrently registered for the half marathon myself. I would run the first leg of the relay for my team, hand off to my teammate, and carry on in the second leg as an individual competitor, completing the half marathon. I was looking to set a personal best and hoped to break the ninety-minute barrier.

My wife and I drove up on the Saturday afternoon in her convertible sports car, enjoying the heat and sunshine of the fading summer. We registered at the hotel, and then I registered myself and my team for the race the next day. When we awoke before the race, one look out the window told us that summer had ended rather abruptly. A driving sleet covered the city. I had only brought racing gear for summer weather, not winter conditions, so I put on my warm-up suit, the red cotton uniform from my Manchester race, and we headed for the start line. The weather wasn't improving as the four team members met at the start line. Two of the runners did have some warmer clothing to help protect from the sleet that was now turning to snow, but Geoff Storms, a six-and-a-half-foot tall plodder, had left the sunshine of Regina that morning in just his shorts and T-shirt, not realizing that he would be facing winter within the two and a half hours it took to make the drive. He wasn't looking forward to running the anchor leg after standing in the cold for three hours.

My teammates all headed to their appropriate meeting points, and I started the race in the snow wearing my floppy warm-up suit that acted like a sail in the gale-force wind and now driving snow. I knew my hopes of setting a personal best had been blown out the window with the winter winds. My only thought now was getting through this ordeal. If I didn't have teammates counting on me, I likely would have gotten back in the sports car, with the top up this time, and driven home. But I persevered and handed the baton to Rick after the first stage and carried on to finish my half marathon in a less than desirable time—out of the prizes, I might add. We three lead runners assembled at the finish line to cheer Geoff as he finished the race for our team. As we saw him plodding to the finish line, we gaped at his long, stocky legs; they were black. At first we thought he had suffered severe frostbite, and then we discovered it was a covering. After he'd left us at the start line, Geoff went to a twenty-four-hour convenience store and bought some extra-large black pantyhose and an extra pair of socks. He cut the feet out of the pantyhose and put them on under his shorts to provide some protection from the elements and put the socks over his hands. He drew lots of stares as he received his congratulations from the grateful teammates. We won the corporate division.

Injuries and Doctors

I have been fortunate to have had far fewer injuries than many other runners. A couple of British runners I ran with regularly in the Middle East attributed that to my late-in-life start to athletics, meaning I didn't suffer all the injuries of young athletes that cause problems later in life. The few injuries I have had made me realize that most doctors don't really understand how to treat healthy people; they are used to dealing with sick people. Their first reaction to any problem is to recommend ceasing your activities. Runners don't appreciate that kind of advice. They want to find a way to keep running, not find an excuse not to run.

I certainly recommend that for serious ailments and injuries, all runners should seek out medical help. However for most minor ailments, a runner is his or her own best doctor. Talking with other runners, reading about sports injuries, or these days doing a Google search will help you through most of your issues without resorting to stopping all activity.

Nutrition

I never have been a fanatic about my diet, but in my forties, and very competitive, I did try to follow the best advice I could find on eating habits. The generally accepted practice was to consume about 60 to 70 percent of your calories in the form of complex carbohydrates—rice, potatoes, bread, pasta—and the remainder in the form of proteins, fruits, and vegetables, with a minimum of fats. I read one book by the nutritionist for Martina Navratilova and other famous athletes and tried to follow his recommendations as much as possible. He based his recommendations on blood composition and had tables on what your ideal blood counts should be and how to adjust your eating to achieve that mix. What I liked best about his plan was that he saw no harm in splurging once or twice a week on whatever you wanted.

I still eat a lot of carbs and try to minimize fats, but I like nothing better than a huge chocolate brownie covered with ice cream and chocolate sauce.

My consumption during a race depends on the type of race and the length of time. During a five- or ten-kilometre running race, I can either get by with no water, or if it's hot, just take advantage of the water stops on the route. For any race less than ninety minutes, I just use water, but if the race will last more than ninety minutes, I like to take on some carbs as they tend to get depleted by the ninety-minute mark. I don't like solid food while racing, but other racers seem to be able to consume sports bars, bananas, and oranges. Sports gels are also quite popular, but I have known people to cramp up from them, especially if they have not trained with them. I just use a simple carb drink, sometimes Gatorade. That seems to be enough to keep me going for my races' two to three and a half hours.

Mental Rehearsal and Visualization

Denard told me early on in my racing life that your IQ drops by at least forty points when the race starts. My bike crash is proof of that; no one in his or her right mind would toss a water bottle overhead while cruising down a steep hill at over seventy kilometres per hour. Helmets are compulsory for the bike ride; my crash was evidence of the axiom I have learned: "If you don't wear one, you don't need one." I know you should wear your helmet on the bike. In one race near Dubai I was on the first lap of the bike portion of an Olympic distance triathlon when instead of squinting into the early morning sunshine I felt a funny sensation with an unusual shade in my eyes. I glanced up and realized that in the transition I had donned my peaked cap for running rather than my bicycle helmet. I was in a panic. This was grounds for immediate disqualification, and I was having a great race so far. The first lap passed by the transition point, where I hopped off my bike, ran into the transition zone, swapped headgear, and remounted my bike to finish the race. No one took note and I won my category, in spite of my detour. Maybe I should have disqualified myself because of my stupidity, but the medal felt good around my neck.

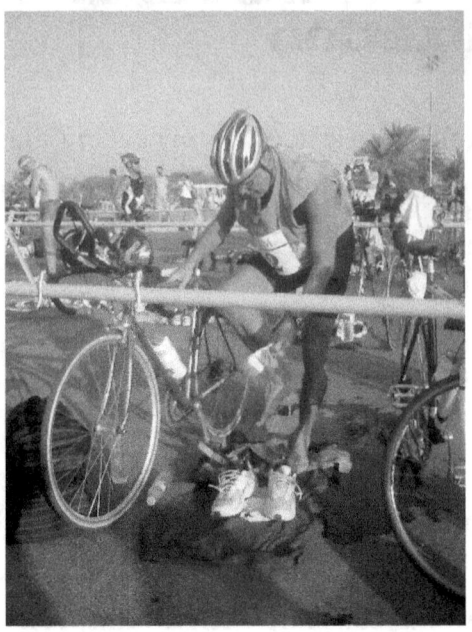

Rushing in the transition zone

One thing I have learned to do is mentally rehearse the race, especially the transition, over and over in my mind. I picture myself coming out of the water, stripping off the wetsuit, donning *all* my bike gear, and starting the ride, changing shoes after the bike and heading out on the run. I continue rehearsing up to race time, carefully laying out all my transition gear where I can access it without thinking, as thinking is not really possible during a race.

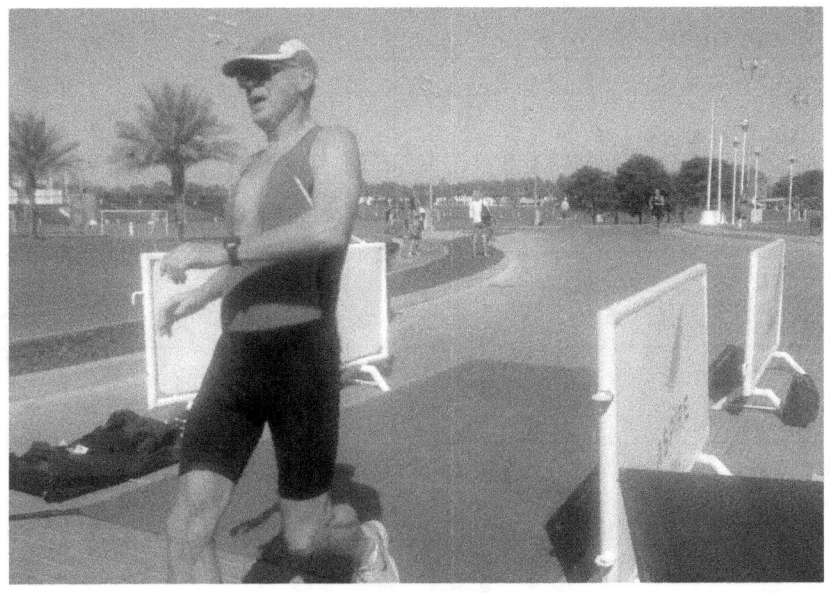

Crossing the finish line

My Personal Bests

Following is a list of my racing times, including my fastest times and most recent races.

Event	Best times		Post-55 best times	
	Time (hr:min:sec)	Age	Time (hr:min:sec)	Age
5 km running	0:18:40	41	0:22:25	60
10 km running	0:38:20	43	0:44:15	56
21 km (half marathon)	1:28: 15	43	1:40:25	57

42 km (marathon)	3:23:10	42	None	
40 km bike time trial	1:00:15	43	1:09:10	60
Olympic triathlon	2:14:05	42	2:29:45	59
Swim (triathlon)	0:25:15	55	0:25:15	55
40 km bike (triathlon)	1:01:20	43	1:06:25	59
10 km run (triathlon)	0:39:20	42	0:47:20	55

My Training Schedule

The following is a typical week of training for me, but not necessarily a prescription for others to follow. I aim for ten hours of training each week with a blend of swimming, running, cycling, and weight training.

Day one
Run—group run, 8 km, 40 minutes
Weights—45 minutes
Total time—85 minutes
Day two
Swim—2,000 metres, stroke drills, 50 minutes
Run—speed work, 12 km, 60 minutes

Total time—110 minutes

Day three

Bike—hill work, 15 km, 60 minutes

Run—hill work, 3 km, 20 minutes

Total time—80 minutes

Day four

Swim—2,000 metres, 100-metre intervals, 50 minutes

Total time—50 minutes

Day five

Run—tempo run, 8 km, 35 minutes

Weights—45 minutes

Total time—80 minutes

Day six

Bike—leisurely ride with friends, 35 km, 90 minutes

Run—LSD, 15 km, 80 minutes

Total time—170 minutes

Day seven

Swim—2,000 metres, 200- to 500-metre intervals, 50 minutes

Bike—speed work, 30 km, 60 minutes

Total time—110 minutes

Weekly totals

Swim—6,000 metres, 150 minutes

Bike—75 km, 210 minutes

Run—46 km, 235 minutes

Weights—90 minutes

Total time—685 minutes (approx. 11.5 hours)

Two things you may notice is that there is no rest day scheduled and the total exceeds my target of ten hours. I never schedule a rest day; at least one of these days disappears due to work or family commitments.

Marathon-Training Plan

The following plan is one that I have used and shared with many others who have embarked on their first marathon. The plan assumes that you are fit and healthy and have a solid year of running behind you. Refer to the information above on the detailed composition of each workout. I have arbitrarily selected the days for the various workouts, but it is not essential to do the activity on those days. Each runner will customise for his or her own circumstances. If you put a checkmark beside each workout that you do, you can monitor your training progress. If your checkmarks equal 80 percent of the total by race day, you should be able to run a comfortable marathon. Most running experts will tell you never to increase your running distance by more than 10 percent each week to avoid injury. This plan attempts to adhere to this rule.

Week	Day	Activity	Quantity	Est. km incl. warm-up and cooldown
1	Monday	Speed	3 times, 1 minute each	8
1	Tuesday	Hills	2 repeats	8
1	Wednesday	Fun run	60 minutes	10
1	Thursday	Tempo	3 km	8
1	Friday	Cross train	40 minutes	0
1	Saturday	LSD		15
1	Sunday	Rest		Weekly total approx. 50 km
2	Monday	Speed	4 times, 1 minute each	10
2	Tuesday	Hills	3 repeats	10
2	Wednesday	Fun run	45 minutes	10
2	Thursday	Tempo	3 km	8
2	Friday	Cross train	45 minutes	0
2	Saturday	LSD		15
2	Sunday	Rest		Weekly total approx. 55 km

	Day	Workout	Description	Distance
3	Monday	Speed	5 times, 1 minute each	10
3	Tuesday	Hills	3 repeats	10
3	Wednesday	Fun run	45 minutes	10
3	Thursday	Tempo	3 km	8
3	Friday	Cross train	50 minutes	0
3	Saturday	LSD		15
3	Sunday	Rest		Weekly total approx. 55 km
4	Monday	Speed	6 times, 1 minute each	10
4	Tuesday	Hills	3 repeats	10
4	Wednesday	Fun run	45 minutes	10
4	Thursday	Tempo	3 km	8
4	Friday	Cross train	50 minutes	0
4	Saturday	LSD		16
4	Sunday	Rest		Weekly total approx. 55 km
5	Monday	Speed	3 times, 2 minutes each	10
5	Tuesday	Hills	4 repeats	10

	Day	Type	Detail	Distance
5	Wednesday	Fun run	45 minutes	10
5	Thursday	Tempo	3 km	8
5	Friday	Cross train	50 minutes	0
5	Saturday	LSD		18
5	Sunday	Rest		Weekly total approx. 55 km
6	Monday	Speed	4 times, 2 minutes each	10
6	Tuesday	Hills	4 repeats	10
6	Wednesday	Fun run	45 minutes	10
6	Thursday	Tempo	3 km	8
6	Friday	Cross train	50 minutes	0
6	Saturday	LSD		20
6	Sunday	Rest		Weekly total approx. 60 km
7	Monday	Speed	5 times, 2 minutes each	10
7	Tuesday	Hills	5 repeats	10
7	Wednesday	Fun run	45 minutes	10
7	Thursday	Tempo	4 km	8

	Day	Activity	Details	km
7	Friday	Cross train	50 minutes	0
7	Saturday	LSD		22
7	Sunday	Rest		Weekly total approx. 60 km
8	Monday	Speed	6 times, 2 minutes each	10
8	Tuesday	Hills	5 repeats	10
8	Wednesday	Fun run	45 minutes	10
8	Thursday	Tempo	4 km	8
8	Friday	Cross train	50 minutes	0
8	Saturday	LSD		24
8	Sunday	Rest		Weekly total approx. 60 km
9	Monday	Speed	3 times, 3 minutes each	10
9	Tuesday	Hills	5 repeats	10
9	Wednesday	Fun run	45 minutes	10
9	Thursday	Tempo	3 km	8
9	Friday	Cross train	50 minutes	0
9	Saturday	LSD		26

				Weekly total approx.
9	Sunday	Rest		65 km
10	Monday	Speed	4 times, 3 minutes each	10
10	Tuesday	Hills	5 repeats	10
10	Wednesday	Fun run	45 minutes	10
10	Thursday	Tempo	5 km	8
10	Friday	Cross train	50 minutes	0
10	Saturday	LSD		28
10	Sunday	Rest		Weekly total approx. 65 km
11	Monday	Speed	5 times, 3 minutes each	10
11	Tuesday	Hills	6 repeats	10
11	Wednesday	Fun run	45 minutes	10
11	Thursday	Tempo	6 km	10
11	Friday	Cross train	50 minutes	0
11	Saturday	LSD		30
11	Sunday	Rest		Weekly total approx. 70 km

12	Monday	Speed	6 times, 3 minutes each	10
12	Tuesday	Hills	6 repeats	10
12	Wednesday	Fun run	45 minutes	10
12	Thursday	Tempo	7 km	10
12	Friday	Cross train	50 minutes	0
12	Saturday	LSD		32
12	Sunday	Rest		Weekly total approx. 70 km
13	Monday	Speed	1 km, 2 repeats	10
13	Tuesday	Hills	6 repeats	10
13	Wednesday	Fun run	45 minutes	10
13	Thursday	Tempo	8 km	10
13	Friday	Cross train	50 minutes	0
13	Saturday	LSD		34
13	Sunday	Rest		Weekly total approx. 75 km
14	Monday	Speed	1 km, 3 repeats	10
14	Tuesday	Hills	6 repeats	10

14	Wednesday	Fun run	45 minutes	10
14	Thursday	Tempo	9 km	11
14	Friday	Cross train	50 minutes	0
14	Saturday	LSD		36
14	Sunday	Rest		Weekly total approx. 80 km
15	Monday	Speed	1 km, 4 repeats	10
15	Tuesday	Hills	6 repeats	10
15	Wednesday	Fun run	45 minutes	10
15	Thursday	Tempo	10 km	12
15	Friday	Cross train	50 minutes	0
15	Saturday	LSD		38
15	Sunday	Rest		Weekly total approx. 80 km
16	Monday	Speed	1 km, 5 repeats	10
16	Tuesday	Hills	6 repeats	10
16	Wednesday	Fun run	45 minutes	10
16	Thursday	Tempo	10 km	12

16	Friday	Cross train	50 minutes	0
16	Saturday	LSD		40
16	Sunday	Rest		Weekly total approx. 85 km

You are now four weeks from your race—time to start tapering

17	Monday	Speed	1 km, 6 repeats	10
17	Tuesday	Hills	4 repeats	10
17	Wednesday	Fun run	45 minutes	10
17	Thursday	Tempo	3 km	8
17	Friday	Cross train	50 minutes	0
17	Saturday	Easy run		10
17	Sunday	Rest		Weekly total approx. 50 km
18	Monday	Speed	1 km, 2 repeats	8
18	Tuesday	Hills	3 repeats	8
18	Wednesday	Fun run	45 minutes	10
18	Thursday	Tempo	2 km	8
18	Friday	Cross train	50 minutes	0
18	Saturday	Easy run		10

				Weekly total approx.
18	Sunday	Rest		Weekly total approx. 45 km
19	Monday	Speed	1 minute, 3 repeats	8
19	Tuesday	Hills	2 repeats	8
19	Wednesday	Fun run	45 minutes	8
19	Thursday	Rest		
19	Friday	Cross train	40 minutes	0
19	Saturday	Easy run		5
19	Sunday	Rest		Weekly total approx. 30 km
20	Monday	Speed	1 minute, 3 repeats	5
20	Tuesday	Hills	2 repeats	5
20	Wednesday	Rest		
20	Thursday	Light run	3 km	3
20	Friday	Rest		0
20	Saturday	Light run	3 km	3
20	Sunday	Race day	Enjoy—have fun	26.1 miles = 42 km

Feel free to contact me at:
brianborgford@hotmail.com